Also by Gill Rapley and Tracey Murkett

*Baby-Led Weaning: The Essential Guide to Introducing
Solid Foods and Helping Your Baby to Grow Up a
Happy and Confident Eater*

*The Baby-Led Weaning Cookbook: 130 Recipes
That Will Help Your Baby Learn to Eat Solid Foods—
and That the Whole Family Will Enjoy*

Baby-Led Breastfeeding

Follow Your Baby's Instincts for Relaxed and Easy Nursing

GILL RAPLEY and TRACEY MURKETT

THE EXPERIMENT

New York

BABY-LED BREASTFEEDING: *Follow Your Baby's Instincts for Relaxed and Easy Nursing*

Copyright © Gill Rapley and Tracey Murkett, 2012

The Photo Credits on page 295 are a continuation of this copyright page.

The Experiment, LLC
260 Fifth Avenue
New York, NY 10001–6408
www.theexperimentpublishing.com

Originally published in the United Kingdom in 2012 by Vermilion, an imprint of Ebury Publishing/Random House Group. This edition, which has been adapted and revised for North America, is published by arrangement with Vermilion.

Many of the designations used by manufacturers and sellers to distinguish their products are claimed as trademarks. Where those designations appear in this book and The Experiment was aware of a trademark claim, the designations have been capitalized.

The Experiment's books are available at special discounts when purchased in bulk for premiums and sales promotions as well as for fundraising or educational use. For details, contact us at info@theexperimentpublishing.com.

Library of Congress Cataloging-in-Publication Data

Rapley, Gill.
  Baby-led breastfeeding : follow your baby's instincts for relaxed and easy nursing / Gill Rapley and Tracey Murkett.
      p. cm.
  Includes bibliographical references and index.
  ISBN 978-1-61519-066-9 (pbk.) -- ISBN 978-1-61519-164-2 (ebook)
  1. Breastfeeding. I. Murkett, Tracey. II. Title.
  RJ216.R334 2012
  649'.33--dc23
                        2012024388

ISBN 978-1-61519-066-9
Ebook ISBN 978-1-61519-164-2

Cover design by Alison Forner
Cover photograph © Marieke Kern

Manufactured in the United States of America

Distributed by Workman Publishing Company, Inc.
Distributed simultaneously in Canada by Thomas Allen & Son Ltd.

First published September 2012

10 9 8 7 6 5 4 3 2 1

Dedicated to the memory of Tracey's mother, Ivy, and her sister, Sally, who both championed breastfeeding long before Tracey had the chance to discover why.

Contents

Part II: What Happens with Baby-Led Breastfeeding

Part III: Less Common Situations

Introduction

BREASTFEEDING IS IMPORTANT. It protects against illness, promotes optimal development, and helps build a strong and lasting bond between mother and baby—laying the foundation for a lifetime's good health and emotional well-being. As evidence grows about how much breastfeeding matters, and research reveals more about the potential health risks of *not* breastfeeding, more mothers are choosing to give it a go. It's the natural and normal way to feed a baby, and it should be an enjoyable and fulfilling experience for both mother and baby.

However, you are likely to come across an enormous amount of conflicting advice and information about breastfeeding from friends and relatives, on websites, and in books—and even from health professionals. Much of this advice (and the outdated practices still common in some hospitals) actually makes breastfeeding *more difficult*. Separating a mother from her baby, imposing parent-led routines, and taking a rigid approach to feeding positions can all interfere with the way a woman's body produces milk and lead to painful and stressful breastfeeding.

As a result, three quarters of babies in the United States start off breastfeeding, but by the end of the first week, half of them have already been given formula. In some states, fewer than a quarter of all babies are having any breast milk at all by the time they are six months old. Many mothers stop breastfeeding before they planned to and many are bitterly disappointed. But the root of most of the common problems is the same—they're caused by struggling against the baby's instincts.

Baby-led breastfeeding is based on how breastfeeding *really* **works**—how your baby's innate skills, his instinct to feed at your breast, and your natural mothering hormones combine to make breastfeeding effective and how, if you let him, your baby will help your body respond to his needs. It works *with* those skills and instincts, rather than fighting against them.

This book explains why following your baby's lead makes sense and shows you how to let him use his instincts to help you breastfeed. It will give you the information and practical tips you need to enjoy relaxed and stress-free nursing, whether this is your first baby, you've struggled with breastfeeding in the past (or are having problems now), or you've only ever used formula. And it will give you the know-how to breastfeed for as long as you and your baby want—whether you stay home or go back to work or school.

Baby-Led Breastfeeding is the book we wish we'd had when our babies were little. Between us we made all sorts of mistakes and encountered a variety of problems. Our experiences since then, as a health professional (Gill) and as voluntary breastfeeding counselors (both of us), have convinced us that babies really do know what they're doing and that responding to them is the key to getting breastfeeding to work. We hope this book will give you the confidence to trust your baby and follow his lead, so that breastfeeding is happy and rewarding for you both.

NOTE

Throughout the book, when referring to the baby, we have alternated between *he* and *she*, chapter by chapter, to be fair to both sexes. And although the information is relevant for both fathers and mothers, we've addressed the reader as the mother, for ease of understanding.

Part I

The Basics of Baby-Led Breastfeeding

1

Thinking About Breastfeeding

BABY-LED BREASTFEEDING IS all about allowing your baby to use his instincts and understanding how you can help your body respond to his needs, so that you can both enjoy easy, stress-free breastfeeding.

There isn't really much you need to do in terms of preparation, and in a sense, you don't even have to make a decision to breastfeed beforehand, because if you are led by your baby he will instinctively want to feed from your breast. However, it can help to know why breastfeeding is considered so important. This chapter aims to provide you with some of those facts, plus some tips on what to expect and what you can do in advance to help things go smoothly.

Is Breast Really Best?

Breastfeeding is the biologically normal way to feed human babies. All babies are born with the instinct to do it and all mothers have milk in their breasts by the time their baby arrives. So it seems a bit odd to talk about the *benefits* of breastfeeding. We don't talk about the benefits of breathing clean air or drinking clean water—we talk about the *risks* of breathing polluted air or drinking dirty water. So it's more accurate to talk about the risks of *not* breastfeeding.

Because of advances in formula manufacturing, these risks aren't as big as they were; but they're there, even so. And a growing amount of research means that we now know more about them, and they're getting harder to ignore.

Most people know that breast milk contains everything a baby needs and that it's always at the right temperature. But there's a lot more to it than that. Research shows that whether babies have breast milk or formula really does make a difference—not just while they're babies, or children, but throughout their lives, whether their parents are rich or poor, wherever they live in the world, and whatever their family medical history.

ILLNESSES THAT ARE MORE COMMON IN BABIES AND CHILDREN WHO WERE FORMULA FED

- gastroenteritis (vomiting and diarrhea)
- necrotizing enterocolitis (a very serious infection of the gut, which occurs mainly in premature babies)
- chest infections and wheezing conditions
- eczema
- middle ear infections
- urinary tract infections
- sudden infant death syndrome (SIDS, also known as crib death)
- leukemia

AND WHEN THEY GROW UP . . .

- obesity
- high blood pressure
- high cholesterol levels
- diabetes

It's not just a question of coughs and colds but serious conditions, such as diabetes and leukemia. The box on page 4 lists illnesses for which there is good evidence of a link with formula feeding as a baby.

The secret lies not so much in the nutrients in breast milk (which can be mimicked reasonably well in formula), but in its other ingredients (which can't). Breast milk protects babies partly through live antibodies, which protect against infections, and partly through factors that support the baby's immature organs, helping them mature quickly and function well, and making them more resistant to disease. The action of feeding at the breast is also important: A breastfed baby's mouth develops differently from the mouth of a baby who is bottle fed. Not only are breastfed babies less likely than formula-fed babies to get infectious illnesses, they're also *more* likely to have straight teeth.

AMAZING ANTIBODIES

Breast milk contains antibodies that protect the baby from infections the mother has had (or been immunized against) in the past, such as rubella (German measles). But her body is also continually making new antibodies as it detects germs in the air around her and in her food—and it sends them straight to the breast, to be added to her milk. So her baby is protected the very next time he feeds. This continual updating is a bit like a computer's virus checker, and it means that breastfed babies are much less likely to catch common infections, such as colds, flu, and tummy bugs—as well as more serious illnesses—than are babies who are not breastfed.

Breastfeeding Isn't Just Good for Babies— It's Good for Mothers, Too.

Women who *don't* breastfeed have a greater chance of developing breast and ovarian cancers than those who do. Breastfeeding seems to help reset the mother's metabolism, too, allowing it to return more easily to the way it was before pregnancy, resulting in higher calcium levels (reducing the chance of osteoporosis and hip fractures in old age) and effective insulin production (which makes the development of diabetes less likely). Breastfeeding also helps the womb return to its nonpregnancy size (see page 22) and has a contraceptive effect (see page 142).

Of course, breastfeeding doesn't *guarantee* good health, but it does make it more likely. And *not* breastfeeding doesn't always lead to illness—but it does increase the risk. The more breast milk your baby has, and the longer you breastfeed, the greater the health protection you both gain. If you are going back to work or school, this means you're less likely to need time off because one of you is sick. Giving nothing but breast milk for the first six months, and continuing to breastfeed well beyond your child's first birthday, is the way to maximize the advantages for both of you.

> "I love the feeling that this child is growing big and strong and beautiful because of what I'm doing—it's all my milk. I know I'm giving him the best start that I can."
>
> Becky, mother of Jack, five months

It's Not Just About the Milk

In the same way that *breast milk* is about more than nutrition, *breastfeeding* is about more than satisfying hunger. The breastfeeding relationship is special, personal, and unique—different for every mother and baby. It gives babies much more than food.

Nursing involves close contact. This closeness means that you and your baby are communicating throughout every breastfeeding, even if you don't say a word. Your nipple and your baby's mouth are both very sensitive, with lots of nerve endings, and your baby is near enough while he's feeding to hear your heart beating. Together, you pick up even the slightest movements and mood changes in each other. Of course, you can hold your baby very close while bottle feeding—but it's not an intrinsic part of feeding in the way it is with breastfeeding.

Breastfeeding mothers and their babies are attuned to each other on a deep biological level. In fact, a nursing mother and her baby are sometimes referred to as a dyad—two individuals so closely linked they are considered one unit. Her body nourishes him; his feeding determines her milk production (see page 209). He relies on her for food; she relies on him to keep her breasts producing milk without becoming uncomfortably full.

Most people know it's important for mothers and babies to bond and that breastfeeding can play an important role in this. A strong bond between mother and baby makes the baby feel secure and loved, and ensures that his mother cares for him. Bonding isn't unique to breastfeeding—formula-fed babies bond with their mothers, too. But because of the hormones it triggers (see "The Role of the 'Love' Hormone," page 22), breastfeeding provides a shortcut to bonding.

Bonding is not only good for babies' development and happiness; it also makes parenting easier. The hormones of breastfeeding make a mother want to respond to her baby and help her interpret his needs. And because it provides pretty much everything a healthy newborn could want (apart from a clean diaper!), breastfeeding makes parenting less stressful and tiring than it would otherwise be.

A breastfeeding mother who is following her baby's lead can often sense when he is going to want to feed—and she doesn't need to decide whether he's hungry, thirsty, or just a bit miserable, nor how much milk to give. She can also offer him a quick snack now and then, to help her fit his feedings around her other commitments. This level of flexibility doesn't happen easily with formula feeding.

Research also shows that nursing mothers get more restful sleep than those who bottle feed, especially if they keep their baby near them at night. This isn't just because the baby doesn't have to wait for the feeding to be prepared; it's because the hormones of breastfeeding are designed to make both of them feel relaxed and drowsy, helping them go back to sleep quickly.

Finally, let's not forget that—when it's going smoothly—breastfeeding *feels* nice! Most mothers find it soothing. Some say it gives them a warm glow. Others say it makes them feel relaxed and slightly spaced out. This feel-good factor is a natural part of breastfeeding and the special closeness that it brings.

> "I find breastfeeding really enjoyable—I love the feeling of Evie being on my breast, the close physical contact, and her lying in my arms. She's almost three now—hopefully she'll have memories of being close to her mom when she was little."
>
> Maria, mother of Evie, 2 years

Why Doesn't Everyone Breastfeed?

Although most people now know that "breast is best," in many Western countries—including the United States—formula feeding has become the usual way to feed babies. A key reason for this is that the advice many mothers are given about how to breastfeed actually makes it more difficult. Feeding schedules, supplementary feeds, and putting babies in a separate room are still recommended by many health professionals, and yet these practices are almost guaranteed to prevent mothers from making enough milk for their baby. As a result, for many generations now women have resorted to formula, believing they can't breastfeed. In addition, many parents today don't live close to their extended family so, even in families where breastfeeding is usual, many children grow up without ever having seen it done. All of this means that knowledge about breast-feeding is no longer passed down through the generations in the way it once was and formula feeding is often taken for granted.

Will I Be Able to Breastfeed?

Many women worry whether they have the right type of breast (or nipple) for breastfeeding. **The size and shape of your breasts will only affect how you hold your baby for feeding—they won't make any difference to how much milk you produce.** It doesn't matter, either, whether your nipples are large, small, prominent, flat, or inverted (tucked inward instead of pointing outward), because babies don't feed by sucking on the nipple; they take a big mouthful of breast (see "Getting the Angle Right," page 34). Gadgets on the market designed to help nipples stand out are for cosmetic purposes only—they aren't necessary for breastfeeding.

Although all kinds of nipples and breasts will "work" for breast-feeding, the following circumstances may mean things are slightly less straightforward:

- *Pierced nipples* don't usually cause a problem with breastfeeding. Occasionally, nipple piercings cause some of the milk ducts to seal over, so milk can't get out from those sections of the breast.

If this happens, milk production will stop in those areas and the rest of the breast will produce more. You should remove any rings or bars before you feed, though, so they don't hurt your baby's mouth, or you may prefer to let the holes close and have your nipples repierced later.

- *Implants* (to increase the size of the breasts) are inserted behind the milk-making tissue, so they don't interfere with milk production or with the baby's getting milk out. Some women who have had implants find that their breasts are a bit tight, making them uncomfortable very quickly if feeding is delayed. You can prevent this by encouraging your baby to feed frequently and by hand expressing your milk whenever he has a longer gap.

- *Breast surgery* can affect breastfeeding, depending on the reason for the operation and the way it was carried out. Surgery to remove a breast lump usually causes damage to the ducts, but only in one area of the breast. The rest of the breast (and the other breast) will work normally. After a mastectomy it's usually possible to fully breastfeed from the remaining breast. However, you should check with your surgeon about whether the reason for the surgery, or any other treatment it involved, might mean that breastfeeding is not advisable.

- *Breast reduction* usually relies on removal of fat tissue (rather than milk-making tissue), but sometimes it involves cutting the milk ducts and the nerves that supply the nipple. If your nipples have been resited—and especially if they are no longer sensitive—breastfeeding may be difficult. Surgery to alter the shape of the nipples can have the same effect. However, breastfeeding *can* work after surgery, and even if you can't breastfeed your baby fully, he may be able to have some of your milk. (A useful website for information on breastfeeding after surgery is www.bfar.org.)

How Do I Prepare?

There are a few things you can do while you're pregnant to get ready for breastfeeding. Taking some time to learn how breastfeeding works and how you can help your baby follow his instincts, and preparing a birth plan that allows you *both* to do this from the very beginning (e.g., by having skin-to-skin contact right away and keeping your baby with you day and night; see Chapter 4) may help you feel more confident. Meanwhile, thinking about how a new baby will fit into your family will make things easier for all of you. If you plan to go back to work or school, try to arrange as much time off as you possibly can—however you feed your baby, the later you go back, the easier things will be for both of you.

Spending time with mothers who are enjoying breastfeeding can be helpful. It's also good to be ready for any stories of breastfeeding failure you come across, from friends, family, or in the media, which can be demoralizing. Almost all women *can* breastfeed—but the wrong advice, especially early on, is sometimes all it takes to make it very difficult. An understanding of what your baby needs to do, and respect for his and your instincts, will help you decide which suggestions are going to be helpful and which may lead to problems.

> "All the way through my pregnancy Paul went on about, 'When life gets back to normal . . .' I don't think either of us realized life would never be the same again. I had more of an idea than him, though—he really wasn't ready for it!"
>
> Anna, mother of Joseph, 20 months

HOW YOUR BODY PREPARES FOR BREASTFEEDING

As soon as you become pregnant, your body starts to get ready for breastfeeding. For many women, tender breasts—caused by the changes happening inside them—are the first sign that a baby is on the way. Here's what's going on:

- The network of blood vessels that supplies your breasts is expanding, helping them prepare for milk making. Some of these blood vessels may show through your skin, giving an effect known as marbling.
- The milk-producing cells in your breast (see page 209) are multiplying rapidly. If you've had a baby before, a few of the cells you made in that pregnancy will still be there—but mostly it's a whole new batch.
- You'll notice your nipples and areolas (the dark skin around your nipples) gradually getting darker and more sensitive—and your nipples may stand out more.
- You may notice small bumps on the skin around your nipples. These are glands called Montgomery's tubercles. They produce an oil that keeps the skin clean and supple and has a smell unique to you, which will help your baby recognize you and trigger his instincts for feeding.
- From about 16 weeks of pregnancy your breasts will start to produce colostrum, a thick, sticky fluid that looks a bit like honey. This is concentrated breast milk (see "The First Milk," page 26). It may leak or form a dry layer on the tips of your nipples, or you may be able to squeeze a bit out. Or you may not be aware of it at all.

Anticipating a Change in Lifestyle

Some people imagine that breastfeeding is very time consuming. This is true in the early weeks, while you are both learning, when it can take more time than bottle feeding. However, as mother and baby get more skilled it becomes quicker and easier, and from about six weeks onward (sometimes earlier), breastfeeding is much less hassle than using formula.

Whichever way you feed your baby, the first few weeks are a period of huge adjustment. Many expectant women find it hard to imagine just how much their baby will need them and how urgent his needs will be, day and night. When a baby needs his mother it's impossible for him to wait patiently, even for a few minutes, because he only understands the way he feels *now*. Some of the things you currently take for granted (such as being able to spend an hour cooking a meal) may benefit from a bit of rethinking so that you'll be able to interrupt what you're doing easily to feed him.

Breastfeeding will work best if you keep your baby close to you, especially in the first few hours and days, and let him lead the way. It's important that your main supporter (whether that's your partner, your mother, or a close friend) understands how much this matters and the difference it will make to how easy or difficult you find breastfeeding. He or she will have a crucial role to play in protecting you and your baby from other people who may—with the best will in the world—want to suggest things that could interfere with your chances of problem-free nursing.

Preparing Your Breasts—What You Need to Do (or Not)

In the past (and sometimes still today), women have been told they should do certain things to their breasts toward the end of pregnancy to get them ready for breastfeeding. They have been advised to toughen up their nipples, to do "exercises" (or wear devices called breast shells or nipple formers) if their nipples are inverted, and to express a little milk now and then to clear out the ducts. All of this has been shown by research to be unnecessary. In fact, a mother's breasts prepare perfectly well for breastfeeding all by themselves (see box).

Rubbing your nipples or applying strong ointments may be harmful, causing pain and damaging sensitive skin. You don't need tough nipples to breastfeed and there are no treatments or creams that will prevent you from getting sore—only attention to how your baby feeds can do that (see Chapter 3).

It *is* a good idea, though, to avoid using soap on your breasts and anything that could make your skin extra sensitive or mask your natural smell (e.g., perfumed bath products) toward the end of your pregnancy.

Expressing colostrum during pregnancy can be a useful way to learn how to hand express (see page 87)—or to reassure yourself that your breasts are doing what they're supposed to (and that your nipples really do have holes in the ends!)—but it isn't necessary and it won't affect your ability to breastfeed. The exception to this is if you know your baby is going to be born early, or if you have a condition such as diabetes (see page 66). In that case you may want to express and freeze your colostrum from about 36 weeks of pregnancy onward, in case your baby needs extra when he's born. Every time you express colostrum, more is made, so there's no need to worry that you'll use it up.

What to Buy—Or Not

Although it can be tempting to buy lots of equipment for your new baby, there's really very little you need for breastfeeding—nature has equipped you with the most important items. There are some extras, though, that may make life easier.

Do I Need a Breastfeeding Bra?

You don't have to buy special nursing bras for breastfeeding, and if you don't normally wear a bra, there's no reason to feel you have to buy one just because you're planning to breastfeed. However, your breasts will be heavier than usual at times (including while you're pregnant), so you may welcome some extra support. A bra is also useful for holding breast pads (see page 79).

It's best to get yourself properly fitted, especially if you have large breasts. Around 36 weeks of pregnancy is a good time to do this, because your breasts will have done most of their growing but your rib cage won't yet have expanded fully, so the bra should fit well when you no longer have a bump. Badly fitting bras can squash the milk ducts and may cause them to become blocked.

Wearing a bra at night will allow you to wear breast pads if leaking is a problem. Nighttime feeding bras are usually light and stretchy with no hook fastenings at the back, making them comfortable to sleep in.

TIPS ON BUYING BRAS FOR BREASTFEEDING

- Make sure the bra fits well, with enough space in the cups to allow for some expansion when your breasts are full.
- If you're buying a bra near the end of your pregnancy, make sure you're not using the tightest fastening already.
- Avoid bras with tight edges that could press into your breasts and squash some of the ducts.
- Underwired styles are best avoided, at least until after the first few weeks, when your breast size will be less changeable.

(continued on next page)

- Go for cups that open fully, so your baby's access to your breast isn't restricted.
- Wide straps are more comfortable than narrow ones if your breasts are heavy.
- If possible, choose a style that's easy to unfasten and refasten with one hand.
- Choose cotton bras; synthetic fabrics will prevent your skin from breathing.
- Expect to need at least three bras, to cope with leaks (especially in the early weeks).

Do I Need Special Clothes?

There are special clothes you can buy for breastfeeding, such as tops with hidden openings and breastfeeding shawls, but there's really no need to purchase any of these unless you want to. Ordinary loose-fitting tops can usually be lifted up with one hand without exposing too much flesh, enabling feeding to be discreet if it needs to be. (Tight-fitting tops can encourage leaking and tend to show off breast pads.)

If you're worried about displaying your postpregnancy "jelly-belly" when you lift your top, you may want to buy a breastfeeding tank or nursing top that has a second, shorter layer of fabric underneath the main T-shirt. This layer stays in place over your tummy when the outer layer is lifted. Alternatively, you can create something similar by wearing a low-cut tank underneath a loose top—just pull the loose top up and the tank down for feeding. Another option is to wear maternity pants or leggings with a high waistband that comes up to your breasts, covering your stomach.

If you want to cover up when you are feeding outside the home, a simple burp cloth over your shoulder or a loose-fitting cardigan or scarf pulled around you may be the easiest solution. Whatever you decide, after a little practice you'll probably find you can breastfeed without anyone seeing what you're doing.

What Equipment Do I Need?

If you're planning to breastfeed, you don't really need many of the baby-feeding products aimed at expectant parents. Although most women find breast pads and burp cloths useful, it's probably best to wait until your baby arrives before buying other things.

If you're going back to work, you may want bottles and perhaps a breast pump, but you won't need them right away—and if you wait until you're ready to express, you may get a better feel for which models will suit your needs. Many women find they don't need to express milk, or that it's just as quick—and more effective—by hand. You may assume you need to buy pacifiers, but they can seriously interfere with breastfeeding in the early days (see pages 37 and 75), so are best avoided for at least the first few weeks.

Some mothers find breastfeeding pillows useful, but one size doesn't fit all, and using a pillow in the early days may prevent you and your baby finding the most comfortable position for nursing (see page 45). Experimenting with a normal bedroom pillow or with different types of breastfeeding pillows (maybe at a breastfeeding group or at a store) once your baby is born will help you decide, but many mothers find that a bunched-up cardigan or baby blanket is more flexible, cheaper, and easier to carry around.

A sling (or baby carrier) is probably one of the most useful pieces of baby equipment, but it's worth waiting until your baby arrives to buy one. That way you can experiment with friends' slings or those in stores to find out which style works best for you—especially if you want to be able to feed your baby while you're "wearing" him.

"I love the freedom breastfeeding gives me compared to bottle feeding. I'll just put him in a sling, shove a diaper, spare onesie and a burp cloth into a little bag and that's all we need. My friends doing formula always seem so weighed down with stuff."

Nicky, mother of Charlie, 5 months

KEY POINTS

- Almost all women can breastfeed.
- Breastfeeding can help your baby resist infections and diseases throughout his life. Not breastfeeding carries health risks for your baby, and for you.
- The more you breastfeed, and the longer you do it, the greater the health protection for you and your baby.
- Breastfeeding isn't just about nutrition—it can make parenting easier.
- A lot of conflicting advice is out there about breastfeeding. Take time to learn how breastfeeding really works and why letting your baby lead the way makes sense.
- Make sure your partner and family understand how breastfeeding works, too, so that they can support you.
- All sizes and shapes of breasts work for breastfeeding. You don't need to do anything special to get yours ready.
- Breastfeeding bras should be fitted when you are around 36 weeks pregnant. Avoid tight edges and noncotton fabrics.
- It's usually better to buy pumps and bottles once you know what will suit you and your baby—you may not need them at all.
- Trying out different slings and pillows once your baby is born is the best way to figure out what you need.

2

How Milk Production Works

BABY-LED BREASTFEEDING MEANS helping your breasts work naturally. Understanding how milk production works will help you get breastfeeding going well from the beginning, so that your baby has the nourishment she needs and your milk supply keeps pace with her changing appetite. It will also help you get things back on track, if you have run into problems. This chapter explains how breast milk is made and how frequent feeding and keeping your baby close will help you make as much as she needs for as long as she needs it.

What Your Breasts Look Like Inside

Understanding the structure of your breasts can help you get them to work well for you so that breastfeeding gets off to a good start. Whatever your breasts look like from the outside, the inside is pretty much the same for all women—except for the amount of fat. Large breasts contain more fatty tissue than smaller ones do, not more milk-making tissue—so size doesn't matter when it comes to breastfeeding.

Here's what your breasts look like inside:

Under a microscope, the milk-making tissue looks a bit like bunches of grapes. Each "grape," or alveolus, is a cluster of

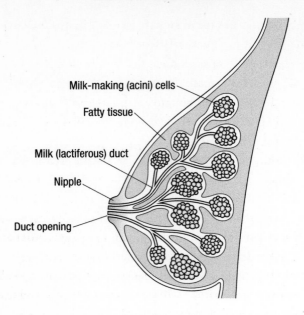

Milk-making (acini) cells

Fatty tissue

Milk (lactiferous) duct

Nipple

Duct opening

milk-making cells called acini cells. The acini cells make milk by taking the ingredients for breast milk from your bloodstream and combining them in the right proportions. The "stems" are the tubes, or lactiferous ducts, that carry the milk out of the breast via the nipple.

Getting Your Breasts to Make Milk

During pregnancy, milk production is minimal, with the breasts producing small amounts of colostrum only. This changes immediately when the placenta is delivered. When a newborn baby is placed on her mother's front, with their skin touching ("skin to skin"), she will instinctively move her head and wriggle around to find the breast. This nuzzling triggers the release of a hormone called prolactin into the mother's bloodstream. Prolactin is detected by a sensitive area on each milk-making cell, and it has the effect of activating or "priming" them. **Skin-to-skin contact between mother**

and baby is a crucial factor in switching on milk production— even if the baby doesn't actually feed right away.

The brain also has sensitive areas that detect prolactin. When these are stimulated they make the mother want to protect her baby and hold her close. This combination of *your* instinct to keep your baby safe and *her* instinct to find your breast makes sure she has access to the milk she needs.

If lots of milk-making cells are activated, your breasts will be able to respond effectively and quickly whenever your baby needs more milk. This means you'll have plenty of milk as she grows and be able to meet her need for extra quantities when she has an appetite spurt (also known as a growth spurt or hunger spurt) or is teething or sick. A milk-making cell that is primed soon after birth will keep producing milk for as long as it's needed, but any cells that haven't been fully primed will start to shut down—and they can't be reactivated until the next pregnancy. Breasts that have only a few active cells are set up for minimum milk production only, so they won't be able to respond when the baby needs extra milk.

Holding your baby skin to skin as soon as she's born and continuing to hold her and allow her to feed as much as you can in the first two weeks will help you activate the maximum number of milk-making cells, so that you can continue to make as much milk as she needs for as long as you want. And if you have two babies, there'll be twice the stimulation, so twice as many cells will be primed.

If you and your baby can't be together during the early weeks (if one of you is sick, for example), getting milk production up and running will be more challenging, but it's certainly not impossible. See page 195 for information on how to make sure your breasts get stimulated even if your baby isn't able to help. On page 224, you'll find information on how to start breastfeeding later, even if you've started your baby on formula.

The Role of the "Love" Hormone

When a baby and her mother are close to each other, another important hormone, oxytocin, is released into the mother's bloodstream. Oxytocin is often referred to as the "love" hormone. It's responsible for:

- making you fall in love
- helping you get pregnant (by making you feel relaxed so you lie down after an orgasm)
- making your womb contract during labor (and afterward)
- helping you fall in love (or bond) with your newborn baby
- making your milk available to your baby

When a baby suckles at her mother's breast, huge bursts of oxytocin are triggered, causing the little muscles that surround the milk-making cells and the ducts to contract. This squeezes the milk down the ducts and is called the let-down reflex, or the milk ejection reflex. If the reflex is very strong, milk may leak (or even squirt) out of the nipples (see photo 6 in the photo insert). **It's a combination of this let-down reflex and the squeezing action of the baby's tongue (see page 30) that allows her to get milk.** In the first week or so, the let-down reflex is a bit erratic and may not happen for a minute or two after the baby starts suckling. However, it soon settles down so that it coincides with the beginning of each feeding.

Some women feel their let-down reflex as a pinching or tingling sensation inside their breasts. Many also say that it gives them a nice drowsy feeling, helping them relax and focus on their baby. Some describe it as being like the relaxed feeling they get after an orgasm (not surprising, really, when the same hormone is responsible for both). So oxytocin not only helps mothers feed their baby, but it makes caring for their baby more pleasurable and less stressful as well.

In the early days, women often feel after-pains (a bit like period pains) when their let-down reflex happens. This is oxytocin making the womb contract, helping it get back to its nonpregnant size and reducing blood loss. (Mothers who are not breastfeeding get after-pains, too—but not necessarily when they're feeding their baby.) This connection between oxytocin, the womb, and the breasts can sometimes work when you don't expect it—for example, making your breasts tingle, and even leak, when you're making love.

BREASTFEEDING CAN MAKE YOU SLEEPY

Breastfeeding is no more tiring than bottle feeding, but the effects of oxytocin can make you want to curl up and snooze. This is useful at night but it may be a bit unexpected during the day. You can either go with the flow and have a nap while your baby sleeps (which is really what your body is telling you to do), or shake off the sleepy feeling by getting up and moving around.

Production on Demand—How It Works

A breastfeeding mother's breasts are never truly empty; breast milk is being made constantly, so there is always something there for the baby, even when she has just fed. However, the rate at which milk is made varies. If the breast is full or if there are long gaps between feedings, production slows down; if the baby feeds more often or drains the breast more effectively, milk making speeds up.

All of this happens because breast milk contains something called the feedback inhibitor of lactation (FIL). The amount of FIL is dependent on the amount of milk in the breast, and its function is to reduce production when it seems the milk isn't needed. So if your baby is feeding infrequently or has had a longer than usual gap between feedings, your milk-making cells will respond by slowing down. But if she feeds frequently, your breasts will carry on producing milk at a steady rate. Nursing two or more babies means the breasts are almost never allowed to get full, so production is maintained at a high rate. More feeding means more milk.

After the first few weeks, FIL and the amount of milk in your breasts (rather than simply how often your baby feeds) are what control how quickly more is made. **If your baby isn't removing milk effectively when she feeds, your milk production will slow down even if she goes to the breast frequently.** See Chapter 6 for information on making sure her breastfeeding is effective.

STRESS WON'T DRY UP YOUR MILK

Women are sometimes told that being stressed can make them "lose their milk." This isn't true. Stress may delay your let-down reflex, so your baby has to wait for a few minutes for your milk to start flowing, but *it's only if feeding is not effective or frequent enough, or if you supplement with formula, that you will start to make less milk.* Page 152 has some tips for helping your reflex work if it's a bit slow.

The FIL mechanism works separately in each breast. This means each breast will make only as much milk as it is asked to make. Some babies feed more on one breast than the other, or even feed exclusively from one breast. When this happens, FIL makes sure that the other breast doesn't keep producing milk that isn't needed (and which would make the mother uncomfortable on that side). Much later, when breastfeeding is coming to an end, it's FIL that helps milk production decrease gradually and comfortably.

The way FIL works means that, *as long as your milk-making cells have been activated,* you can increase or decrease milk production on demand. If your baby needs more milk, nursing her more frequently will put in the order for extra to be made. There will be a delay of a few feedings, but you'll soon notice production increasing. The same thing applies in reverse: If feedings get further apart, production slows down—but again, it will take your breasts a while to adjust.

It's all about telling your breasts what's needed.

HOW TO MAKE SURE YOUR BABY GETS ENOUGH MILK

The best ways to be sure your baby gets all the milk she needs:

- Let her feed whenever she wants.
- Let her feed for as long as she wants each time she nurses.
- When she finishes feeding on the first breast, *offer* her the second (but don't worry if she turns it down).

This is the essence of baby-led breastfeeding. Feeding this way will ensure that your baby gets the nourishment she needs and that your milk production keeps pace with her changing appetite. It is also more likely to lead to easy, pain-free nursing than following a predetermined schedule or routine is.

How Breast Milk Changes to Meet Your Baby's Needs

Breast milk changes during the course of a single feeding and throughout the day. It also changes as the baby gets older to meet her growing needs.

The First Milk

The first milk produced by your breasts is called colostrum. It's usually yellowish and sticky—a bit like clear honey. Colostrum is a concentrated version of breast milk. It's packed with important nutrients and antibodies to nourish your baby and protect her from infection, and it comes in small quantities, for some very good reasons.

Once she's born, your baby needs to learn how to coordinate sucking and swallowing with breathing; colostrum allows her a couple of days to practice this new skill before she has to cope with larger volumes of milk. At the same time it allows her kidneys to adapt gently to life outside the womb, and her stomach—which is tiny at birth—to expand and adjust gradually to taking in more milk.

Over the first four or five days, your milk will become less concentrated as other ingredients (especially water) become part of the recipe. If your baby is allowed to feed frequently, she'll gradually be able to manage larger feedings as the volume of milk increases. But if she doesn't feed often, she may well find the amount of milk—and the strong flow—difficult to cope with. There's also a good chance that your breasts will become overfull, leading to engorgement (see page 243). Offering your baby the chance to feed when you feel your breasts becoming full will help prevent discomfort for you while keeping the flow manageable for her.

It used to be thought that colostrum lasted for only three days—until the "real milk" came in. In fact, pretty much all the ingredients of colostrum, including the antibodies that protect against disease, continue to be made. Colostrum is special because it is so concentrated, which is what a newborn baby needs. Later milk is less concentrated but is just as nutritious and protective as colostrum.

"MY BREAST MILK IS ORANGE!"

The color of breast milk changes over the first few days, usually becoming creamy-white or white. It's not unusual for there to be a small amount of blood in the milk (caused by the normal increase in blood flow to the breasts in the first week or so), so that it appears pink or orange. This is known as "rusty pipe syndrome." Later, other colors are possible, too: Some mothers say their milk looks bluish, while others find that eating a lot of leafy vegetables gives their milk a green tinge. All of these variations are normal (but see page 238 for more on blood in breast milk).

Breast Milk Changes During a Feeding

Once the colostrum-only stage is over, the composition of your milk will change gradually during each feeding. The first few mouthfuls from each breast are quite watery—a sort of drink or soup course—with lots of nutrients but not much fat. Then the amount of fat begins to increase, with the milk getting progressively fattier through the main course to the dessert. The more watery milk is sometimes referred to as "foremilk" and the fatty milk as "hindmilk," but these terms are misleading. There aren't two sorts of milk and there isn't a single point during the feeding when the milk changes from one type to the other. It just gets gradually creamier (and higher in calories) with every mouthful.

Breast Milk Changes over a Day

Your breast milk will vary slightly over the course of a day. For example, when your baby has just finished feeding, the milk remaining in that breast will be very fatty, but within a few minutes it will start to become more watery again. The rate of milk production will also vary; most mothers say they produce more milk in the morning than in the evening.

Some research suggests that milk produced in the evening is higher in fat than that produced earlier in the day and that night-time milk contains a natural sleep-inducing chemical that calms babies and helps them fall asleep. Whether or not this is true, breastfeeding at night has a soothing effect on both mother and baby (see page 23).

Breast Milk Changes as Your Baby Gets Older

Your breast milk will continue to change as your baby gets older. Your breasts will adjust the ingredients very slightly all the time, in line with her growing needs, and the antibody content will vary according to the infections your body detects around you (see "Amazing Antibodies," page 5). Then, as breastfeeding gradually winds down, your milk will become more like colostrum again. This is because a child who isn't feeding often but is out in the big wide world, exposed to lots of germs, needs concentrated shots of protective antibodies, just as she did when she was newborn.

Your Baby Knows What She Needs

Breast milk can be food or drink—or both. Sometimes your baby will want a quick drink, so she'll just have a few mouthfuls of milk from one breast. If she's really thirsty, she may come off the first breast and want a couple of sucks from the second as well. On another occasion she'll want a "three-course meal" from one breast and a "drink" from the second—or she may decide to stay on the second breast for longer, so that she gets second helpings of all three courses. Sometimes she'll even want to go back to the first breast again! All of this is quite normal.

Babies don't need any other drinks, even in hot weather. In fact, giving babies even small drinks of water can fill their tummy and dull their appetite for milk, reducing their resistance to illness and possibly limiting their weight gain. The breasts reset themselves very quickly between feedings in terms of the fat/water balance, so a new feeding will always be thirst-quenching. **Your baby is the only one who knows what she needs—you can trust her to get the right balance of food and fluid when she feeds.**

KEY POINTS

- Skin-to-skin contact with your baby and frequent feeding activate your milk-making cells.
- The more often your baby nurses early on, the more milk you can make long term. Milk production can then be stepped up or down later, according to your baby's needs.
- When your baby suckles, oxytocin—the "love" hormone—triggers your let-down reflex, which sends your milk down the ducts toward the nipple.
- Feeding whenever your baby wants will ensure you keep making plenty of milk. If you let your breasts get too full, milk production will slow down.
- Breast milk starts off as colostrum, which is packed full of nutrients and protective ingredients. It becomes less concentrated over the first few days as the volume increases.
- Breast milk can be food or drink, or both. It gradually changes throughout a feeding, from watery (thirst-quenching) to creamy (full of calories).
- Breastfeeding works best when it's baby led.

3

How to Breastfeed

BABIES HAVE A natural instinct for breastfeeding and don't need to be taught what to do. However, they do need the opportunity to figure out how to do it, and they need plenty of practice in the beginning to get good at it quickly. Baby-led breastfeeding is about trusting your baby's abilities and allowing plenty of time for him to learn. It's about holding him in a way that makes it easy for him to feed, and being aware of things that could make breastfeeding more difficult for him. Following his lead means he will get the milk he needs, and you will avoid many common problems.

This chapter explains how your baby attaches to the breast to feed, what he has to do to get milk out of your breast, and what you can do to help him become skilled at breastfeeding.

The Secret of Pain-Free Feeding—Attachment

The secret to effective, pain-free breastfeeding lies in the attachment between the baby's mouth and the breast. To get lots of milk, your baby's mouth needs to be full of breast, so he can squeeze the milk from the ducts easily. And to feed without hurting you, he needs to have your nipple right at the back of his mouth, where it can't be damaged.

To get the milk out your baby will use his tongue and lower jaw in a combination of "yawning" and squeezing. He'll open his mouth wide (like the baby in photo 23), scoop up a large mouthful of breast and nipple, and make a secure seal with his lips. Then he'll:

1. drop his lower jaw in a yawning movement (without breaking the seal), to allow the ducts to fill with milk;
2. raise his jaw again, trapping some of the milk in the ducts;
3. use his tongue to press the breast against the roof of his mouth, squeezing the trapped milk out of the nipple into the back of his mouth;
4. swallow the milk.

He'll repeat this cycle over and over, in a rhythmic way, while he's feeding.

If your baby has hold of just the nipple and a small amount of breast:

- He'll lose his grip easily when he tries to drop his lower jaw.
- There won't be much milk available for him to squeeze out.
- Your nipple will be pinched against his hard palate.
- He'll have to suck hard to keep the nipple in his mouth.
- He'll get tired long before he's had a satisfying feed.
- Your breast won't be effectively drained and your nipple may get damaged.

The result could be, for you:

- sore nipples
- engorgement
- mastitis
- a slowing-down of milk production

And for your baby:

- frustration
- exhaustion
- constant hunger
- slow weight gain

Sometimes a baby can seem to be nursing well at the beginning of a feeding, when the mother's let-down reflex (see page 22) is at

BREASTFEEDING IS DIFFERENT FROM BOTTLE FEEDING

Many people assume that breastfeeding is like drinking from a bottle with an artificial nipple, but it's very different. Here's why:

Put the end of your thumb into your mouth and give it a few sucks. Notice how much of your tongue is in contact with your thumb and how it moves against it. This is like bottle feeding. Now put your thumb right in—up to the second joint—and suck it again. This is like breastfeeding.

When your thumb is deep inside your mouth, much more of your tongue is in contact with it, so you can use your tongue to squeeze it against the roof of your mouth. The tip of your thumb is free, up by your soft palate (the squashy bit at the back) where there's more space. And you don't have to keep sucking to hold on to it.

This is why your nipple needs to be in the back of your baby's mouth when he breastfeeds. If he tries to feed as if he is sucking from a bottle, your nipple will be squashed; it will be harder for him to keep it in his mouth and he won't get enough milk. He needs a good mouthful of breast *plus* nipple to feed effectively.

its strongest. But once the reflex subsides and the milk flow slows down, if he isn't effectively attached he won't be able to get big mouthfuls of milk and he'll become frustrated or tired. If this is repeated every time he nurses, his mother's breasts will have more milk left in them than they should, and they'll get the message that less is needed.

Your Baby Knows How to Breastfeed

Babies have a strong instinct to breastfeed. They are born wanting to find the breast and they go through a very distinctive pattern of behavior to help them do this (see page 54). Recognizing your baby's instincts—and allowing him to use them—will give him the best chance of breastfeeding effectively.

When they are near the breast, babies bob their head around and use their hands in a kneading action to orientate themselves and figure out how best to approach the nipple. This behavior is a crucial part of the feeding because it allows babies to get to the breast and position themselves so that they can attach easily. It will happen more quickly as your baby gets more skilled, but it's important that he isn't disturbed or hurried if he seems to be taking his time during the first few weeks.

When he can feel or smell that he is near his mother's nipple, a baby will naturally start to open his mouth and stretch his tongue forward. This is known as rooting and it's part of his preparation for scooping up the breast to feed. **Once he's figured out where the nipple is, he'll tip his head back. This helps him open his mouth really wide and come to the breast chin first.** It also means that, if the nipple was roughly level with his nose beforehand, it will now be near his top lip and pointing toward the roof of his mouth. All of this helps him get a really good mouthful of breast, with the nipple touching his soft palate.

Working with Your Baby—"Latching On"

The moment when a baby attaches to his mother's breast is sometimes known as latching on. It's a crucial part of breastfeeding, but it usually happens in less time than it's taken you to read these two sentences. One minute, your baby is bouncing his head against your breast, and the next, he's taking his first gulp. Blink and you'll miss it. What happens during these few seconds—and whether or not your baby attaches successfully—depends on whether his mouth and your breast can make contact easily.

Getting the Angle Right

Your baby needs to scoop up your breast with the nipple pointing toward the roof of his mouth, rather than straight on, because otherwise his tongue will get in the way. The space for your breast is in the *upper* part of his mouth, not the middle. (If you put your finger into your own mouth, first centrally and then pointing upward, you'll feel how high up the space is.) If your nipple goes into your baby's mouth centrally, he won't be able to draw it deep inside, so he won't get much milk (and he may make you sore). Photos 15 to 17 show a baby scooping up the breast at just the right angle.

Mothers are sometimes told they need to make sure *all* the areola is in their baby's mouth when he feeds. This isn't true. The areola is just a part of your skin and most areolas are too large to fit inside a baby's mouth. **What is important is that, if your areola is an even shape, with the nipple in the middle of it, when your baby is feeding you should be able to see more of your areola above his top lip than below his bottom lip** (as in photo 18).

To achieve this angle, your baby needs to tip his head back and come to the breast with his chin leading. He will do this instinctively, provided nothing stops him. However, any sort of pressure on his head—even just a finger—will prevent him from tilting his head back and will push his nose (rather than his chin) into your breast. Not only will this make it difficult for him to attach and feed, it may also make him cross and lead to him "fighting" at the breast. Depending on his position, you may need to support your baby's neck and shoulders—but try to avoid holding his head, so that he can tip it back easily (see "How Should I Hold My Baby for Feeding?", page 39).

Getting the Timing Right

If you are lying back with your baby on top of you, gravity will help him attach, so you won't need to do very much at all. He'll attach himself when he's ready—as the baby in photos 20 to 24 demonstrates. If you're holding him in another position, you'll need to be ready to bring him closer to your breast at just the right moment. This means moving him quickly toward you (*not* pushing your breast toward him), when his mouth is at its widest. Babies tend not to hold their mouth open for very long, so the best moment for latching on only lasts a second. If you miss it, just ease your baby away and start again.

If your baby's first attempt to attach doesn't result in a large mouthful of breast, he'll probably let go and try again, opening his mouth a little wider this time. However, some babies are reluctant to open their mouth really wide, usually because they haven't learned that this is what they need to do. If your baby attaches without scooping up a good mouthful of breast, he probably won't get much milk and he is likely to make you sore.

If your baby doesn't seem to want to open his mouth wide, express a drop of milk so he can smell it on your nipple, or touch it to his lips so he can taste it. If this doesn't tempt him, rub his nose gently against your nipple and then move him away. A brief light touch, repeated several times, will be more effective than simply holding him with his nose against your breast. Keep "teasing" him like this—without letting him attach—until he opens his mouth really wide.

THAT OUCH! MOMENT

You may experience an "ouch" moment at the beginning of feedings in the first few days while you and your baby are getting your positioning and timing sorted out. This shouldn't last more than about ten seconds. If it does, try pulling his bottom closer to you; if that doesn't work, just take him off your breast and start again. (Slip a finger into the corner of his mouth to break the suction before easing him away gently, so that you don't damage your nipple.)

Sometimes babies become agitated and end up sucking their fists instead of the breast, as though they're confused about what they should be doing. This is normal behavior. Sucking has a soothing effect, so sucking his fists helps a fretful baby calm down. And moving his hand between the breast and his mouth also helps him find exactly where the nipple is. Focusing on relaxing *yourself* and talking gently to your baby will help him relax and figure out what he needs to do.

What Makes Latching on Difficult?

The most likely reason babies find it difficult to attach (or latch on) to the breast is that they are not being held in the most helpful way (see page 39 for information on holding your baby for feeding). Another common reason is that the breast is overfull, making it difficult to scoop up. In this case, hand expressing a little milk (see page 87) will soften your breast and make it easier for your baby to manage.

Overfull breasts are often the result of a long gap between feedings—and a long gap can mean a very hungry baby. Being overly hungry is stressful, and this can make it difficult for the baby to relax and let his instincts guide him (especially if he has been crying), so he struggles to attach effectively. This makes the baby more stressed and can easily lead to a vicious cycle, where feeding is painful for the mother and frustrating for them both.

Nursing whenever your baby wants to, and offering him the opportunity to feed as soon as you notice your breasts feeling full—even if he's asleep—should prevent him getting too hungry *and* keep your breasts from becoming uncomfortable. It will also give him plenty of opportunity to fine-tune his technique.

Long or very wide nipples can occasionally make latching on difficult because they trick the baby into starting to suck before he's scooped up enough of the breast. If your baby is struggling to get a big enough mouthful because you have large nipples, you may be able to help him by gently pressing your thumb into your breast *just above your baby's nose* to tilt the nipple up slightly as you offer it to him, then let it unfold into his mouth. This will help him scoop up more than just the nipple. It will also exaggerate the angle at which the nipple points inside his mouth, helping him draw it in deeply before he starts sucking.

A baby who has a tongue tie (see box) may also find latching on difficult.

Bottles and Pacifiers Can Interfere

A baby doesn't need to scoop up the nipple of a bottle (or a pacifier). In fact, he only needs to open his mouth a little way and someone will put it in for him. Many babies who have been given a bottle or a pacifier while they are learning to breastfeed subsequently make only half-hearted attempts to open their mouth, or they latch on to the nipple alone, instead of the breast. This doesn't

WHAT IS A TONGUE TIE?

In babies with tongue tie, the frenulum, which joins the tongue to the floor of the mouth, extends farther forward than usual. This extra membrane restricts the movement of the tongue and prevents the baby from scooping up and compressing the breast effectively. He may slip off the breast easily, feed very briefly, and ask to feed again after only a few minutes. He's also likely to get frustrated and tired at the breast—and his mother may develop sore nipples. A tongue tie can make bottle feeding difficult, too.

A tongue tie is sometimes easy to see, because the tip of the baby's tongue makes a heart shape when he tries to stretch it forward, but it isn't always obvious. Some babies who appear to have a tongue tie can breastfeed without a problem. Others can be helped to attach effectively if the mother tilts her nipple upward (by pressing gently with her thumb opposite the baby's nose) as her baby scoops up the breast. Feeding positions where the baby is more upright can also help (see photos 21, 30, and 34).

It's important that tongue tie is diagnosed early so that the mother and baby can get help with breastfeeding. Some babies need their frenulum to be cut or "divided," which is usually quick and painless, with the baby being handed straight to his mother afterward for a feeding. (Older babies are inclined to wriggle, so they may need an anesthetic.) If your baby seems to be finding breastfeeding difficult, contact someone with expertise in breastfeeding (see "Where Can I Get Help?," page 108) as soon as you can.

always happen, but it's impossible to predict which babies will react like this, so if you do plan to introduce a bottle, it's best to avoid it for a few weeks until your baby has gotten the hang of breastfeeding (see "Getting Breastfeeding 'Established,'" page 111).

Nipple Shields Rarely Help

Nipple shields are sometimes recommended for mothers whose nipples are flat or inverted, or when babies are having difficulties attaching to the breast. These soft silicone devices are worn over the nipple and areola during breastfeeding.

However, just like a bottle, they can be poked into a baby's mouth and can make it *appear* as though the baby is feeding well. In reality, many babies will struggle to accommodate a shield *and* scoop up the amount of breast they need to feed effectively. And they will learn to expect the shield, meaning it can be difficult, later, to persuade them to feed without it.

Nipple shields may also cut down the amount of stimulation the breasts get while the baby is feeding (leading to reduced milk production). Some mothers who have a tendency to produce more milk than their baby needs (see page 219) *may* be able to feed with a nipple shield long term, but for most women they are best avoided.

How Should I Hold My Baby for Feeding?

A lot of books and leaflets about breastfeeding give detailed instructions involving special chairs, pillows, footstools, and ways to hold the baby. All of this can make breastfeeding much more complicated than it needs to be. Time spent getting yourself and your baby into exactly the "right" position for feeding is likely to make him frustrated and unable to latch on easily, so feeding becomes unnecessarily stressful for both of you.

Every woman is built in a unique way. Your body proportions, breasts, and nipples are different from other women's. You may have a tender cesarean scar or perineal stitches that affect how you can position yourself and your baby. And, of course, each baby is different, too. All these things affect how you will hold your baby for feeding—which means that it's difficult for anyone to predict exactly what you'll need to do without knowing a bit about you and your baby.

YOUR BODY SHAPE MAKES A DIFFERENCE

Your body shape will influence the way you need to hold your baby for feeding. Look in a mirror: Notice how your breasts hang and which way your nipples point (sometimes referred to as your "angle of dangle"!). A mother with small, pert breasts will need to hold her baby much higher up her body than will a mother whose breasts are large and pendulous, with downward-pointing nipples, and her baby will need to face her in a slightly different way. It's quite likely, too, that your right breast hangs slightly differently than the left one, so be prepared to adjust the way you hold your baby when he swaps sides. There's no standard breastfeeding position—you'll soon find what works for you and your baby.

It's Your Baby's Position That Matters

The way you sit, stand, or lie at the start of a breastfeeding doesn't really matter, provided you're reasonably comfortable—what matters is how *your baby* is positioned. This is what will determine whether he can breastfeed effectively, without causing you pain. (To understand why, try drinking a glass of water with your head turned sideways. Or ask someone to put a hand on the back of your head, to stop you from tipping it back while you drink. How easy is it for you to open your mouth, tip your glass, and swallow if your neck is twisted or you can't tip your head back? It's no different for your baby.) Once he's feeding, you can move around and adjust your own position (see page 45), if you need to.

Babies (especially older ones) can feed in all sorts of positions, as photos 25 to 34 show. But for a position to work it must allow your baby to use his hands to help him, to tilt his head back easily, and to scoop up your breast with your nipple pointing toward the roof of his mouth.

ESSENTIALS FOR HELPING YOUR BABY FEED

For your newborn baby to be able to attach and feed effectively, he needs to be:

- close to you, with as much of his body in contact with yours as possible (check for gaps—his chest and hips should be touching you; pull his bottom in close)
- his whole body in line (i.e., with his knees facing the same way as his nose)
- his body weight supported (neck, shoulders, and hips)
- his head and arms free to move
- his nose lined up with your nipple ("nose to nipple")

These factors are important, however you hold your baby for feeding; they happen automatically in some positions but can easily be overlooked in others.

Lying Back Can Be a Good Way to Feed

One of the easiest positions for a baby to learn to breastfeed is lying on his tummy, with his mother half sitting and half lying, supported by pillows or cushions (see photos 20, 21, 25, and 34). This is sometimes known as the laid-back or Biological Nurturing™ position. This position is easy for your baby because:

- He is close to your breast, so he doesn't have to stretch (and you aren't tempted to lean forward and give yourself backache).
- Your breast is underneath him, so gravity helps him attach and stay attached (rather than pulling him away, as it would do if you were more upright).
- He is facing your breast, so he doesn't have to twist awkwardly.
- He can lift and turn his head freely, using his arms to help him balance.
- He can change his position to bring his nose into line with your nipple (so that when he tilts his head back, the nipple will be aiming at the roof of his mouth).
- His whole body is in contact with you, so he feels safe.
- You don't have to support his weight with your arms.
- You don't have to judge when he is ready to attach or help him by bringing him to your breast at the right moment.
- You can trust him to position himself, rather than feeling that you have to get everything "right."

The first breastfeed happens like this for many babies (see Chapter 4), and it's the position that will make best use of your baby's feeding instincts when he is new. Many mothers also find it easier because all they have to do is to stop their baby falling sideways— which makes it especially useful for feeding twins. (You'll need to adapt it slightly after a cesarean section, though—see page 62.)

Nursing this way allows your baby more control than being held in your arms and gives him a better chance of learning how to feed effectively. This will make it easier for him to adapt to other feeding positions later. However, nursing like this doesn't need to be limited to when your baby is young or while he is learning to breastfeed—a child of any age can feed this way. It's especially useful in the evenings, when many babies want to have lots of feedings close together, because it allows you to simply lie back on the couch with your feet up while your baby "helps himself."

> "It took me months before I realized I didn't have to feed my baby cradled in my arms. A friend told me she fed lying down—I couldn't believe it! So then I fed like that a lot—even during the day, sometimes on my side and sometimes with me on my back on pillows and Rachael on my chest. And when she was big enough, I'd sit on a chair and she'd just have a quick feeding standing up!"
>
> Michelle, mother of Rachael, 4 years

tip

If you're supporting your baby's neck and shoulders with your hand, watch that your fingertips and thumb don't creep up the edges of his ears. If they're that high, he won't be able to tip his head back and latch on at the right angle.

There Are No Set Positions for Feeding

Although lying back to feed is great for learning, there will be situations when another position will be more convenient, so it's worth exploring a few options. Lots of books describe specific positions for breastfeeding, but provided it works for you and your baby, in reality anything goes. Whether he's wrapped across your front, tucked under your arm, being carried in a sling, or lying next to you on a bed, the same basic principles apply (see "Essentials for Helping Your Baby Feed," page 41). If what you've chosen is helpful for him, he'll be able to attach to the breast and feed easily. If it's *unhelpful,* he may struggle to get a good mouthful or find it difficult to suck or swallow.

It's easy to be tempted to start off by cradling your baby with his head resting in the crook of your elbow. This position is fine for bottle feeding, but it makes it harder for a breastfeeding baby to nurse effectively in the early weeks. It won't allow your baby to reach the breast comfortably (without twisting), tip his head back, or swallow easily. If you want to cradle your baby in your arms to feed, make sure he's facing your nipple and rest his neck on your forearm instead.

There's no need to aim to have eye contact with your baby while he's feeding. Babies enjoy feeding in a variety of positions—and many feed with their eyes closed. You and your baby will be communicating throughout every feeding through touch and smell, so eye contact isn't necessary.

As you experiment with a few different positions, you'll find one or two that are favorites for you and your baby, but they may not always turn out the way you expected. Don't be surprised to find that:

- When you hold your baby across your front to feed from one breast, most of his body is over by your other breast (as in photos 28 and 32).
- When you hold your baby under your arm to feed (sometimes called the "football" or "clutch" hold; see photos 26 and 33), most of his body is behind you. (You may need to make sure he isn't pushing himself too far forward with his feet.)
- When you lie down on your side to feed (see photo 31), your baby's shoulders are well below your breast. (You may need to straighten your legs until he is attached

and feeding so that he doesn't use your thighs to push himself upward.)

It's worth finding a few different positions that you and your baby like and to vary the way you hold him occasionally, just to help make sure that milk is removed from all parts of your breasts. This will help prevent you from developing blocked ducts (see page 245).

BREATHING WHILE FEEDING

There's normally no need to hold your breast away from your baby's nose while he feeds. If he's been allowed to come to the breast "nose to nipple," and to tip his head back and attach with his chin leading, his nostrils will be free. If a cushion or tight clothing is pushing the breast into your baby's nose, it's better to move what's causing the problem than to press your finger into your breast.

If your baby's nose is buried in your breast, it's unlikely his chin will be pressed into it, which means he hasn't got a good mouthful. Holding the breast away from his nose may allow him to breathe but it won't enable him to feed effectively. It may also prevent some of your ducts from draining properly. He needs to be helped to come off the breast and start again.

Getting Comfortable Once Your Baby Is Feeding

As long as you are holding your baby in a way that allows him to breastfeed easily, how you position yourself is a personal thing. Apart from protecting your cesarean scar (if you have one)— perhaps with a small cushion or rolled-up towel—the best approach is to focus on *your baby's* needs first and figure out what else *you* might need once he's feeding. This will save a lot of time and make life easier for both of you. Don't assume you'll need a pillow to support him—struggling to position your baby *and* a pillow can make things more difficult.

> "When I nursed the twins together I'd often sit cross-legged so I could move my knees to position each baby individually. The football hold worked sometimes, too. But it was nice to nurse them separately as well, so I had a hand free and could move around more easily."
>
> Siobhan, mother of Connor, 4 years,
> and Orla and Sophie, 2 years

Once your baby has latched on and started to feed, think about whether you need to change your position slightly. Wriggle around a bit to get comfortable. If you need to move (e.g., to sit more upright or lean back), hold your baby firmly against your body so that you take him with you as you adjust your position. Provided he was able to latch on easily, and you brought him to your breast rather than moving your breast toward him, his attachment will usually be secure enough to allow you to move without dislodging him. You may want to stuff a cushion, baby blanket, cardigan, or towel under your elbow (to help you support your baby's weight) or in the small of your back. You are the best judge of what needs to be where, so don't be afraid to experiment.

> "Feeding Joe was painful but I'd be too nervous to move him, so I would just put up with it. But with Bella, I take her off if it's not right and once she's on okay I move around to make sure we are both comfortable. I'm much more relaxed and we haven't had any problems so far."
>
> Jackie, mother of Joe, 3 years,
> and Bella, 6 weeks

Do I Need to Hold My Breast?

There's no need to grip your breast while your baby is feeding. He comes to your breast, not the other way around, so it's not necessary to lift your breast up, point it in a certain direction, or try to put the nipple in your baby's mouth for him. Distorting the breast's natural shape can interfere with the instincts that help a baby breastfeed. And having your fingers pressing into your breast during a feeding may prevent your milk flowing properly.

You may find it helpful to steady your breast while your baby is attaching, but unless it's very heavy, you should be able to release it once he has latched on. Some mothers with large breasts find they can see what they're doing more easily if they support their breast underneath and use their thumb to flatten the top slightly, just until their baby is attached. If you're worried that letting go of your breast will make your baby lose his grip, experiment with moving him down a little first, so that the weight of the breast doesn't pull it away from him.

If you have very heavy breasts, you may find you are more comfortable if you support the weight of your breast throughout the feeding. You can use your hand to do it, but that will tend to push your baby away from you and may make nursing difficult for him. It might help to use your other hand to support him so that your breast-supporting hand is out of his way, as in photo 32 (sometimes known as the cross-cradle position). If you find that taking the weight of your breast makes your arm ache, you may find it easier to put a small rolled-up washcloth or burp cloth under your breast, or to use a scarf tied behind your neck as a sort of breast sling. Take care, though, that nothing is squashing or digging into your breast while your baby is feeding.

However you feed your baby, it's important that your clothes don't get in his way (or yours) or stop your breasts from hanging freely. Your bra, if you wear one, should allow you to uncover each breast fully while feeding, so that its shape isn't distorted. If you choose to wear a normal bra instead of a nursing bra, undo it—or slip the strap off your shoulder—for nursing. Just lifting the cup from underneath is not a good idea because the tightness of the bra across the top of your breast could prevent it from draining properly, which in turn could lead to a blocked duct or mastitis. The same thing applies to a bikini top.

Is My Baby Feeding Effectively?

The difference between a baby who is breastfeeding effectively and one who is struggling to get milk is obvious—*if* you know what to look for. However, many people (parents, grandparents, and health professionals) don't realize that breastfeeding is different from bottle feeding. So, when they see a baby sucking strongly (usually with his lips pursed and cheeks drawn in), or notice that his ears are moving, they assume he is feeding effectively. They couldn't be more wrong.

Here's what a baby who is breastfeeding effectively looks like:

- His chin is pressed into the breast (because his head is tilted back).
- He has a wide-open mouth and (although you may not be able to see it) his bottom lip—not his top lip—is curled back, because he attached with his chin leading.
- His cheeks are full and rounded (because his mouth is full of breast).

- More of his mother's areola is showing above his top lip than below his bottom lip (because her nipple is angled up toward his soft palate, right at the back of his mouth). (Note: If your areola is very small, you probably won't be able to see any of it.)
- He sucks and swallows in a rhythmic way (see page 94).
- He lets go of the breast spontaneously when he's had enough (see page 96).

You can see most of these signs in photo 18. Check for them yourself while your baby is feeding. (If you have large breasts and can't easily see your baby's mouth, you may want to use a mirror, or get your partner or a friend to have a look.) If any sign is missing, it's likely that feeding is *not* effective, even if the other signs are present.

Two other signs of effective feeding are important:

- Your nipple should be the same shape and color at the end of the feeding as it was at the beginning (not squashed or pinched).
- Apart from a possible "ouch!" moment at the beginning of the feeding while you are both learning (see page 36), nursing should be painless.

However, pain-free feeding and undamaged nipples don't necessarily mean that all is well. Look for all the signs listed above, just to be sure.

Shutting your eyes occasionally while your baby is nursing will help you learn what effective feeding feels and sounds like, so you don't always need to check what it looks like.

Take Your Time—and Trust Your Baby

Breastfeeding takes time to learn. Even if you've done it before, it will be different with this new baby. And he needs to practice, too. Babies often wriggle around, attach, and let go a few times at the beginning of a feeding, but eventually they find what feels right and settle down to a pattern of rhythmic sucking and swallowing. Latching will get quicker as your baby learns what to do, but in the meantime you'll need to be patient and let him figure things out. If you try to help him by putting the breast in his mouth or holding his head, he's likely to become *more* frustrated, not less, because his instincts are telling him this isn't what's supposed to happen. If you've followed the "Essentials for Helping Your Baby Feed" on page 41, your baby will do the rest.

KEY POINTS

- Ineffective attachment of the baby at the breast is the cause of most common breastfeeding problems.
- Babies have strong instincts to help them breastfeed; your role is to make it easy for your baby to do what he needs to do, not to try to help him by doing it for him.
- Using bottles and pacifiers can interfere with babies' learning.
- Breastfeeding is different from bottle feeding and babies need to be held differently for each.
- A lying-back position can be helpful for learning.
- When holding your baby to nurse, focus on his needs first, then make yourself comfortable once he's feeding.
- Breastfeeding shouldn't hurt. Except for a few seconds at the very beginning of a feeding in the early days, pain while nursing is a sign that something is wrong.
- You and your baby need time to learn—together.

Part II

What Happens with Baby-Led Breastfeeding

4

When Your Baby Is Born

BABY-LED BREASTFEEDING BEGINS at birth. When a baby is born, both mother and baby are already primed with instincts and reflexes, ready for breastfeeding. These natural responses are triggered by skin-to-skin contact between them, and if this is not interrupted, breastfeeding happens naturally. Many mothers who didn't plan to breastfeed have been surprised at how right it can feel to let their newborn baby follow her instincts and feed.

Normal, healthy, full-term babies know how to breastfeed. Their drive to find the breast is at its strongest immediately after birth and gradually weakens in the hours and weeks that follow. This chapter is about how to support your baby to use her instincts and how to make the most of your first precious hours with her—as well as what to do if this can't happen.

Why Skin-To-Skin Contact Is So Important

Skin-to-skin contact is the best way for breastfeeding to start. It's also enormously important for bonding with your baby, to help you both to feel safe and recover from the birth. When your naked baby is against your chest, surges of hormones are created, which tell your breasts to start making milk (see page 20). They also start the process of you falling in love with your baby and wanting to protect her.

For your baby, skin-to-skin contact is the nearest thing to when she was in the womb, so it helps her adjust to being outside your body. Being held skin to skin regulates her temperature; your chest is the warmest part of your body, so it's the best place for her to be to stop her getting cold. Skin-to-skin contact also allows your baby to pick up some of your natural skin bacteria, helping protect her from infections. She will be able to hear your heartbeat and she'll recognize your voice. Your reassuring presence will help steady her breathing and calm her. Just as you did before she was born, as a new mother you can provide everything she needs at this special time.

Skin-to-skin contact triggers the instincts that help babies breastfeed:

- *Crawling to the breast:* Drawn by the unique scent produced by the glands around your nipples (which is similar to the smell of your amniotic fluid), your baby will instinctively press her feet and knees into you and push herself toward your breast. This instinct fades gradually in the first few weeks—by the time she is six weeks old she will have "forgotten" how to crawl.

- *Finding the nipple:* When your baby's head brushes up against your breast she'll spontaneously lift or turn it to find your nipple. Then she'll tilt it back, open her mouth wide, and use her tongue to scoop up a big mouthful of breast. She may wriggle around and bob her head up and down several times before she gets it just right.

- *Starting to suck:* Once she's scooped up a mouthful of breast, your baby will automatically start to suck. And, because she has an innate preference for sweet tastes, she'll love the taste of your milk.

These instincts are strongest in the first hour or two after birth, so if both mother and baby are well this is the ideal time for them to be in skin-to-skin contact.

Your Baby's First Breastfeeding

As soon as your baby is born—even before the placenta is delivered—ask your birth partner and your midwife to help you get comfortable lying back (supported by cushions or a bean bag) with your baby on top of you. You'll need to have your tummy and chest bare (no bra or top), though you may want something around your shoulders if the room is cool.

Your baby should be dried quickly—but not wrapped. With a blanket or towel over her back, she will be safe and warm. Make sure the cover isn't tight or too heavy, so she can move her head and limbs easily. If the room is cool and her hair is damp, ask for a hat for her so that she doesn't lose heat. Photos 1 to 4 and photo 12 show a mother and baby skin to skin, just after the birth.

Let your baby take her time to discover the feel of your skin and your unique smell, and to crawl gradually toward your breast. Expect her to have short bursts of activity with periods of rest in between.

It usually takes at least half an hour—and often an hour or more—for a newborn baby to find her mother's breast and start to feed. There's no rush, though. Babies aren't born hungry; they have been fed through the umbilical cord right up until the point of birth. This first feeding is a way for your baby to discover for herself what she needs to do, so that she knows how to latch on later, when she *is* hungry.

"Jake fed even before the placenta was delivered. The midwife lifted him on to my belly and within minutes he was obviously looking for something. He knew exactly where to go and what he wanted. He started feeding straight away—he just knew what to do. With Beth it was different. I didn't have skin to skin with her. When I offered her the breast she licked it and sniffed it, and nuzzled a bit, but she didn't feed properly for about twelve hours."

Ruth, mother of Jake, 2 years,
and Beth, 6 weeks

It's important that, as far as possible, no one and nothing interferes with your baby's instinctive behavior. She is the one doing the feeding. You may need to support her weight a little, but don't be tempted to help her find your nipple or open her mouth. Her head must be free to move and bob about—it shouldn't be held or pushed on to the breast—and she needs to be allowed to do things in her own time. If she is interrupted before she gets as far as feeding, she will have to start again, right back at the beginning, slowing everything down and delaying her learning.

Letting your baby lead the way from the moment she's born will cement her instincts and make breastfeeding easier for both of you. Rushing her or trying to do it for her can make everything harder.

Giving Your Baby's Instincts a Chance

All new mothers and babies respond in similar ways when they are in skin-to-skin contact, because their hormones and instincts take over. It's important for those around them to help protect this special time and to prevent any interruptions. Others may be rushing about (especially in a busy maternity unit), but these precious moments only happen once for each mother and baby.

Old-style care involved getting the baby into a crib as soon as possible after the birth so that the mother could rest, but as long as you are comfortable and there is someone with you to make sure your baby is safe if you drift off to sleep, having her with you—feeding, nuzzling, or sleeping—will probably help you relax more than being separated from her. This is partly because you'll know she's safe and partly because the hormones triggered by her closeness will help you feel relaxed and sleepy.

Skin contact shouldn't normally need to be postponed or interrupted for your baby to have a routine examination, while the placenta is delivered, or while you have stitches put in. A skilled midwife or obstetrician can examine a baby while she is lying on her mother—and, provided your vaginal area is properly numbed, having your baby to hold can be a good way to take your mind off being stitched. **It's reasonable for you (or your birth partner) to challenge anyone who suggests interrupting your skin-to-skin contact with your baby unnecessarily.**

Aim to stay in skin-to-skin contact with your baby at least until she has had her first breastfeeding. If you have to be moved to a different room before that, ask if you can stay in skin contact during the move. If this isn't possible, start skin contact again as soon as you can—preferably before you have a bath or shower, so that you don't confuse her by changing how you smell.

It's helpful if your partner and other relatives understand in advance why it's so important that only *you* should be holding your baby for the first hours. Everyone wants to cuddle with a new baby as soon as they can, but passing your baby around from one person to another while you and she are still getting to know each other will confuse her and may hamper breastfeeding. For some mothers, just having more than their birth partner in the room is enough to make it difficult for them to really focus on their baby. Let your relatives know this is the best time to get breastfeeding going well and for you and your baby to bond.

What About Newborn Tests?

There are various tests and treatments that your midwife or physician may want to carry out on your baby—and you'll probably be keen to know what she weighs, too. But all of this can mean interrupting your time in skin contact. Most procedures can wait until after the first breastfeeding—especially if you've made it clear in your birth plan that this is what you'd prefer. If weighing can't be postponed—perhaps because the health-care staff need to complete the birth records—then the best alternative is to ask to have your baby weighed *as soon as she's born*. It will only take a few seconds to lift her into the scales and then back onto you—and it will mean she can then take all the time she needs to find your breast and nurse for the first time.

Can My Partner Have Skin Contact?

Skin-to-skin contact is a lovely way for a baby to bond with both her parents, but there are two key reasons why you, as her mother, should be given priority. First, skin contact really is the best way to get going with breastfeeding and it can help you avoid a lot of common problems later. Your baby's feeding instincts will never again be as strong as they are immediately after the birth, so it makes sense to make the most of them.

Second, the first skin-to-skin experience your baby has should be with you because labor and birth are very stressful—and skin contact is the perfect way for both of you to relax, rest, and recover. From your baby's point of view, she's been inside you all this time, so it's *you* she's expecting to meet; she wants to hear your voice and smell your scent—and it's *your* reward for all that hard work.

All of this doesn't mean your partner or birth companion has to be excluded—he or she can hug *both* of you. But at this special time, your supporter's main role is to keep you and your baby together and safe, and to speak up for you both if anyone tries to separate you. This is enormously important because it allows you to focus on your baby and tune in to her needs.

What If My Baby Is Sleepy?

If you have been given pain-relieving injections or an epidural anesthetic during labor, your baby may well be born with some of the drugs still in her system. Her body will deal with this more slowly than yours, and she will probably be quite sleepy—perhaps for a couple of days.

If your baby is drowsy when she's born, it's especially important that her skin-to-skin contact with you is not interrupted until she's had her first breastfeeding. Babies who are sleepy at birth usually take longer to find the breast and start feeding—as much as two or three hours. It may seem as though she is not interested and it can be tempting to put her in a crib to sleep it off. But babies who are sedated by drugs can sleep for many hours, and if they are not in contact with their mother, their instinct to search for the breast can start to weaken. It's not unusual to have problems getting breastfeeding going when this has been allowed to happen, so it's worth insisting on skin-to-skin contact with your baby if you and she are both well enough.

What If Things Are Complicated?

Not all births are uncomplicated, so skin contact and nursing sometimes have to be adapted at first. If the baby has been born very early (or if either the mother or baby is sick), skin-to-skin time may even have to be put on hold (see Chapter 11). But if both are well, it should still be possible even if there have been complications around the time of the birth.

The First Breastfeeding for Twins or Triplets

How ready newborn twins or triplets are to breastfeed depends on how mature they are. Multiples are often born early, and premature babies may need special care following the birth (see Chapter 11). But if they are well enough to be with you, having skin contact with more than one baby shouldn't be a problem, with a little help.

If your babies are born normally, you may have the opportunity to cuddle quickly with the one who arrives first. However, you will need to hand him or her to your birth partner when the second one is ready to be born so that you can concentrate on pushing. Once the birth is over, you'll probably need a little help to position your babies on your tummy and stop them from falling, but that's really the only challenge—they are used to sharing a cramped space.

Like any other babies, full-term multiples can feed themselves, if given the opportunity. They may be ready to feed at the same time, but there's every chance that one will lead the way. Either way, if the babies are well there's no need to rush to get it all to happen quickly.

"After the twins were born I let each baby crawl up to the breast in turn. It was very slow because they were so sleepy but they found their way, latched on and had a feed. When the first was finished I gave her to my husband and did the same with the other one. They were just like little newborn animals—it was wonderful."

Sam, mother of George, 4 years,
and Zoe and Ellen, 2 years

If It's a Difficult Birth

Unless you are sick, or your baby needs special care (see page 191), skin-to-skin contact is the best way for both of you to recover from a difficult birth. However, it's especially important to have someone else there to make sure you are both safe if you are very tired, weak from losing blood, or if an anesthetic has left you drowsy or unable to move much.

Your baby may have bruising and a headache, especially if she was born with the help of a vacuum pump or forceps. This is likely to make her irritable, particularly if her head is handled in an effort to help her feed. Letting her take her time to begin nursing, preferably on top of you, with you in a lying-back position, will mean her head is less likely to be touched.

If being born has been a struggle, it's quite likely your baby will be too exhausted to feed at first. If your midwife or pediatrician feels she needs food quickly, you can express some of your milk for her. Because the first milk, colostrum, is thick and the quantities are small, hand expressing (see page 87) will be much more effective than pumping—and it's easy to do, even if you're lying down. Ask for help if you need it. You can express the milk either

IF YOU ARE OVERWEIGHT

If you are very overweight, you may be more likely to have a complicated birth and experience a delayed start to milk production. Spending lots of time in skin-to-skin contact with your baby and asking for help to find feeding positions that work for you both will give you the best chance of getting breastfeeding off to a good start.

directly onto your baby's lips, onto your fingertip, or, if she needs medical attention, into a small syringe, so she can have it right away. Holding her skin to skin while you express will help your milk flow *and* help her recover from the birth.

After a Cesarean Section

Having a cesarean section doesn't necessarily mean you and your baby can't have skin contact immediately; it all depends on whether you are awake during the birth and how well you both are. As the importance of skin-to-skin contact for all mothers and babies is becoming more widely understood, more hospitals are encouraging mothers who have a cesarean birth under epidural anesthetic to hold their baby this way while the surgery is being finished. Make sure your doctor knows in advance that you would like to have skin-to-skin contact with your baby as soon as safely possible.

Some babies will have their first breastfeeding in the operating room, but operating tables aren't very wide, so the time you spend in the recovery room may be a better opportunity for relaxed and undisturbed skin-to-skin contact. Your birth partner can play a big part in helping you find a comfortable position and hold your baby safely, especially if you are coming round from a general anesthetic. Lying back, with your baby across your upper chest (as in photo 14), or on your side (see photo 31), may be more comfortable than having her on your belly.

Some mothers who have a cesarean section find that their milk production takes a while to get going. Spending plenty of time in skin-to-skin contact with your baby after this type of birth can make a huge difference to your chances of a positive start with breastfeeding.

"Lola was born by C-section and she had skin to skin straight away—she was just laid on top of me and she fed for a good half an hour while I was being stitched. I was the last operation of the day and no emergencies came in so we had plenty of time. Now I usually feed Lola like that first thing in the morning. I lie back on the pillows and she just finds the nipple herself and gets on with it."

Rebecca, mother of Lola, 11 weeks

If You or Your Baby Is Unwell

Sometimes it isn't possible for mother and baby to have skin contact immediately after the birth: for example, if the baby is born very prematurely (see Chapter 11) and needs to go to the intensive care nursery or into an incubator, or if she needs to be given oxygen. Such circumstances may mean that skin contact has to be delayed—but it doesn't mean it can't happen at all. And it certainly doesn't mean that breastfeeding won't be possible.

If skin contact has to be postponed because *you* are unwell, your baby can have it with your birth partner instead. This will calm and comfort her and enable the two of them to begin their own bonding. Meanwhile, hand expressing some colostrum will help kick-start your milk production as well as providing food for your baby (see pages 87 and 194).

If you can't spend time skin to skin with your baby as soon as she's born, be sure to let the hospital staff know that you want to do this as soon as possible and try to make sure that your first breastfeeding together—however much later this is—starts this way. You may also want to discuss ways of feeding your baby in the meantime that will interfere as little as possible with her instincts to breastfeed (see "Feeding Your Baby Before He Is Ready to Breastfeed," page 199).

The First Forty-Eight Hours

The first day or two after your baby's birth can be a bit overwhelming, especially if you are in the hospital. Some hospitals and birthing centers allow partners to stay round the clock, but it's more common for them to be asked to leave, especially at night. So it's a good idea to think ahead about what will make it easier for you to respond to your baby, if there's no one right by you to help.

> "It was hard the first night in the hospital. I lay staring at Maya in her little crib and I kept putting my hand on her to check she was breathing. I was so worried each time she woke up because it meant I had to get her out of the crib and try to feed her. I just didn't have a clue what to do."
>
> Safiya, mother of Maya, 3 months

You are likely to be exhausted in the first few hours after giving birth and you may have drugs in your system that make it unsafe for your baby to stay in your bed. However, you won't want to move far to reach her—especially if you are finding moving difficult, so make sure and tell the staff that you want her to room in with you. You'll also want to be able to wake up quickly when she needs you. Some hospitals are introducing cribs that clip on to the mother's bed, but if that option isn't available (and it's worth asking, just in case), ask your birth partner to help you get your baby's crib as close to your bed as possible so that you can reach her easily and lift her out for feeding (and put her back) with the least effort.

Laying your baby skin to skin on your tummy for feedings will make nursing more instinctive for both of you. It will also avoid your having to figure out how to hold her and how to get the timing right for latching on, because she'll do most of it by herself.

However, if you are sore or have stitches, you may find it difficult to get comfortable. If you're prepared to be creative and can get someone to help you lift her and move pillows or cushions to where you need them, you'll be able to find a position for feeding that works. It doesn't matter if it's unconventional—what's important is how your baby is positioned against your body (see page 40), not whether you are sitting or lying in a certain way. Don't be afraid to ask for painkillers to help you move more easily.

Some women find it difficult to relax and sleep in the day or two following their baby's birth; others feel overwhelmingly tired and are nervous about sleeping too deeply. Don't be afraid to ask a member of staff to wake you if necessary so your baby can nurse, and to come and check on you both later, in case you fall asleep during the feeding.

The best place for your baby (unless one of you is sick) is right next to you—day and night. Insist on keeping her with you, if you need to.

> "I had an emergency C-section with Jacob and we were both traumatized for the first few days. All the time we were holding on to each other it was fine but as soon as we were separated he would start crying—and so would I."
>
> Kelly, mother of Austin, 4 years,
> and Jacob, 2 years

If Your Baby Needs Encouragement to Feed

Not all babies feed frequently on the first day and some have as few as three feedings in the first twenty-four hours. Provided your baby is full term (at least 37 weeks) and has nursed within an hour or two after birth, this shouldn't be a problem. But from the second day onward she should be showing signs of wanting to feed more frequently. If this isn't happening by the time she's a day and a half old (perhaps because she is very sleepy, either recovering from the birth or sleeping off the effects of drugs you were given in labor), or if you feel under pressure to give her formula, it's probably a good idea to start offering her the breast more often—even if she seems to be asleep.

Babies' instincts are so strong that the smell and feel of their mother's breast tends to make them want to breastfeed even if they haven't got the energy to do anything else. Holding your baby skin to skin and expressing a little milk on to her lips may be enough to tempt her to latch on. If not, ask your midwife or nurse for help to give her some expressed milk in a cup or with a syringe.

If You Have Diabetes

If you have diabetes, your baby is likely to need some extra feedings while her metabolism is adjusting to being outside the womb. To avoid her being given formula (which may—according to some research—trigger diabetes later in childhood), you can express and freeze your colostrum toward the end of pregnancy. This can then be given to your baby by cup or syringe, instead of a formula feeding (you may need to explain this to staff who may not be familiar with this practice).

Making sure you have a snack whenever your baby nurses will help keep your blood sugar from dropping afterward.

KEY POINTS

- Uninterrupted skin-to-skin contact as soon as possible after the birth is the best way for breastfeeding to start.
- A lying-back position, with your baby on top of you, will allow her to use her instincts for her very first feeding.

- Your baby knows what to do. Let her lead the way and try not to interrupt her or interfere.
- Relax—it can take an hour or more for a newborn baby to find the breast and start to feed.
- Don't wash your breasts until your baby has fed at least once, so she can recognize your smell.
- Your birth partner can help make sure skin-to-skin contact is not interrupted until your baby has had her first breast-feeding (and for as long as possible after that).
- If skin-to-skin contact can't happen immediately after the birth, it can still happen later.
- Don't be afraid to ask for the help you need in the first few days to care for your baby and hold her for nursing.

5

The First Two Weeks

THE FIRST TWO weeks after a baby's birth are a period of huge physical and emotional adjustment, even for experienced parents. Adapting to a new baby in the family, getting to understand his needs, and recovering from the birth all present their own challenges.

These two weeks are also crucial for breastfeeding. Frequent and effective feeding during this time, and learning how to follow your baby's lead, will lay the foundation for long-term, stress-free nursing and optimum milk production. In many cases where breastfeeding goes wrong, the problem can be traced back to this very early period.

Investing plenty of time at this stage (even if you plan to combine breastfeeding with formula later) will help you avoid the sort of difficulties that so many mothers and babies encounter. This chapter explains how.

Having a Babymoon

The first two weeks of breastfeeding can be thought of like a honeymoon, only with your baby as the focus of your attention. The idea is to concentrate on getting to know him, and on breastfeeding, with as few distractions and other responsibilities as possible. Some people call this a "babymoon."

The essence of a babymoon is spending as much time as you can holding your baby skin to skin. Keeping him against the warmth of your chest, where he can nuzzle your breast and feed whenever he wants, will make the most of his instincts. It will also cause surges of prolactin and oxytocin, triggering milk production and your instinct to nurture him, and making the adjustment to motherhood easier.

A babymoon relies on your partner, family, or friends helping with meals and housework so you can focus mainly on your baby. It doesn't necessarily mean you have to be secluded or stay indoors, as long as you can spend time getting to know him. It works best if you establish a kind of "nest" for you both—maybe in bed or on the couch—that's comfortable and easy for feeding (but see page 118 for safety information). If you have an older child or children, spending time with them will be important (especially if they are still breastfeeding), but your newborn needs to be your priority.

Getting to know your baby can be easier if you don't have lots of people dropping in to visit—especially if you are likely to feel inhibited about breastfeeding in front of them. Limiting visitors for a week or two (or limiting how long they stay) will also prevent your baby being passed around and fussed over, which may tire him out or lead to his feeding cues going unnoticed—especially if whoever is holding him thinks babies don't need to be fed unless they cry. Many new mothers find that a day with lots of visitors leaves them exhausted, with painfully full breasts and a fussy baby who has difficulty latching on. Try to stay near your baby whenever anyone else is holding him, so that you can spot when he needs you and feed him promptly.

A babymoon allows you to get confident with breastfeeding in your own time, without having to worry about who's watching and whether you're doing it "right." This will make it much easier, later on, to nurse your baby when there are other people around and to resist well-meant but unhelpful advice.

> "I had all my visitors on the day I came home and Ben just slept through it, in my arms. After that we didn't see anyone for about ten days. I stayed in my pajamas and the three of us spent a lot of time in bed, with Ben feeding and us gazing at him. It felt like it was our time to knit together as a family—I wouldn't give it back for anything. And by the time people started saying things like, 'Are you sure he's getting enough?,' I was confident enough not to take any notice."
>
> Caroline, mother of Ben, 5 years

It's a good idea to warn your friends and relatives in advance if you plan to limit visitors at first, and explain to them why this is important to you. There will be plenty of opportunities later for them to get to know your baby, but these first two weeks are your best chance to get breastfeeding going well.

Putting In the Order for Milk

The first two weeks of breastfeeding establish your potential for long-term milk production. The more your baby nurses during this time, the more milk you will make now—and the more you will be able to make later, whenever it's needed. **Your breast milk is all he needs unless there is a genuine medical reason for him to be given something else.** Formula or water will fill up his tummy and make him less eager to breastfeed.

Bottles and pacifiers are best avoided, too. A pacifier may make your baby sleep longer than he should or prevent you from spotting that he needs to feed, meaning that feedings are delayed or missed, while giving him anything in a bottle—even your expressed breast milk—may interfere with the way he uses his mouth to breastfeed.

The acronym **FEEDS** is an easy way to remember what's important, especially in the early weeks. To give you and your baby the best start, breastfeeding needs to be:

- *Frequent:* day and night—expect your baby to nurse *at least* eight times every twenty-four hours in the first two weeks (and probably more, especially if some feedings are very short) and *at least* six times every twenty-four hours after that
- *Effective:* with your baby attached so that he can get milk easily
- *Exclusive:* with your baby having only your milk—no other drinks or food, not even water
- *On Demand:* whenever your baby asks—or sooner, if he's sleepy or your breasts are uncomfortably full—and for as long as he wants each time
- *Skin to skin* as much as possible, in the early weeks

"Jude was always a hungry baby and fed a lot. I loved that lazy and relaxed pace of life. I'd spend all afternoon on the couch feeding—it was all about nurturing him. He was born in the ninety-first growth percentile and never lost any weight. He was just getting what he needed."

Anka, mother of Jude, 2 years

Frequent Breastfeeding Is Good for You and Your Baby

Lots of small feedings allow your baby to learn to coordinate his breathing with sucking and swallowing. They also allow his stomach (which is about the size of a marble at birth) to stretch gently. Colostrum, with its highly concentrated nourishment, is the perfect food for the first few days, and if he feeds frequently, your baby will be able to adjust as the volume of milk increases—and he'll keep you from getting overfull.

Frequent breastfeeding in the beginning also makes a difference in how well your baby adapts to life outside the womb. Research shows that, compared with babies who have few feedings, those who nurse frequently from birth:

- lose less weight in their first week
- have less jaundice (see page 84)
- stimulate their mothers to make more milk

Frequent breastfeeding will also:

- prevent you from becoming engorged (see page 243), keeping you comfortable and making it easier for your baby to latch on
- establish your long-term ability to make plenty of milk
- give you and your baby lots of opportunities to practice breastfeeding instinctively, with less time between feedings to forget what you need to do

The frequency of your baby's feedings is likely to reach a peak around the fifth day, when it may feel as though he is *always* wanting milk. After that, things will gradually settle into a pattern, though this will be different for every baby. Some feedings will be long, others just snacks—but you can expect your baby to nurse *at least* eight times a day in the early weeks, and quite possibly twelve times or more.

ADULTS FEED FREQUENTLY, TOO!

Breastfeeding is food *and* drink for babies. If you add up all your own snacks, meals, and drinks, you may be surprised how often you eat and drink. You probably don't eat at regular intervals, or go for very long without a little something, and the amount you consume—and how quickly you do it—will vary each time. You may even find that, except at night, you feed *more* often than your newborn.

"Sometimes Chana used to feed for a while then fall asleep and want to nurse again fifteen or twenty minutes later. She seemed quite happy with it but I was stressed thinking she needed another feeding so quickly. I didn't realize it was probably the *same* feeding. She was having a little break—just as we would in a restaurant before the dessert."

Jazmin, mother of Chana, 16 months

FEEDING ISN'T JUST ABOUT HUNGER

Your baby doesn't have to be hungry or thirsty to want—and need—to nurse. Breastfeeding provides babies with comfort, warmth, and security as well as food and drink—and it's impossible to overfeed a breastfed baby. If your baby is asking to feed and you think he can't possibly be hungry again, you may be right—but that doesn't mean he doesn't need to be offered the breast. Responding to your baby's requests will make both parenting and breastfeeding easier.

Babies need to feed through the night as well as during the day, and night feedings can be as unpredictable as daytime feedings, at least in the first few weeks. Many exhausted new parents find this one of the hardest things to adjust to, but the more practice with breastfeeding you and your baby have during the day, the easier nursing at night will become. Once you don't need to concentrate so much to breastfeed, you won't need to wake up completely or turn the light on to do it at night. (See page 116 for more on nursing at night.)

Understanding Your Baby

Part of getting to know your baby is understanding how he communicates and what he is trying to tell you. In the first couple of weeks, most of his requests will relate to his needs for feeding and security, because survival is his priority. Keeping your baby next to you, night and day, will enable you to know when he wants to feed and make caring for him much easier.

Offering your breast when your baby is only just stirring means he is likely to attach more easily. You'll soon find that your let-down reflex happens before you've even picked him up, which means that he doesn't have to wait for food to be available and learns to trust you to be there when he needs you.

Knowing When Your Baby Needs to Feed

Babies let their parents know that they want to feed through a variety of "feeding cues," but some are very subtle and it's easy to miss them. If a baby is asking to nurse and no one responds, eventually he will cry. **Many people think crying is the only way babies tell us they want to feed, but in fact it is a baby's final attempt to get his message across to someone who can**

help. From the baby's point of view it's all about survival, so his desperation is genuine.

Waiting until a baby cries before nursing makes breastfeeding unnecessarily difficult. Here's why:

- Crying gets in the way of latching on, so it can prevent babies from feeding effectively.
- Crying gives babies gas, which can make them uncomfortable after nursing.
- Crying makes babies stressed, causing them to get frustrated at the breast and making it difficult for them to feed in a relaxed way.

It's not just the baby who gets stressed if his cues are ignored. Listening to a baby cry, even for a few minutes, is stressful for the adults around him. It's *supposed* to be like this because it's an alarm to warn the mother her baby needs her. Answering your baby before he gets upset will help him feel safe and make feeding easier.

Recognizing when your baby needs to nurse involves watching and listening to him carefully, especially while you're still getting to know each other. His first signals are likely to be very brief or subtle (see box). If he is not offered a feeding fairly quickly, he will become more active until eventually, if he's still ignored, he will start crying.

Some babies are very sleepy for several days after birth (see page 59) and don't get past the murmuring stage (see box on the following page) before going back into a deep sleep. It's especially important for someone to recognize these very subtle cues, so the baby doesn't miss out on the chance to nurse.

Pacifiers can prevent some feeding cues, such as sucking movements, from being spotted. And some babies will find a pacifier so soothing that they drift back off to sleep without anyone knowing that they needed to feed. Long gaps between feedings send messages to the breasts to slow down milk production, which can mean the baby doesn't get enough milk to put on weight.

Keeping your baby close will allow you to spot his earliest feeding cues. The sooner you notice that he wants to nurse, the more chance you'll have to finish what you're doing or get yourself a drink before he starts to get upset, so that you can settle down for a relaxed feeding. Carrying him in your arms or in a sling, or having him lie beside you in bed at night (see page 117), will mean you feel his smallest movements and get the earliest possible signal that he would like to feed. At night, this will give you a chance to wake up enough to nurse him without either of you needing to be fully awake.

Letting your baby lead the way means not making him wait to feed—but it doesn't mean you always have to wait for him to ask. If you become engorged, you'll be in pain and he'll find it hard to attach. So, if your breasts feel uncomfortably full, it's in your baby's interests as well as yours to offer him the chance to feed a bit earlier than he'd planned.

EARLY CUES THAT YOUR BABY WANTS TO FEED

- moving his eyes under his eyelids
- moving his head and stretching his neck
- making gentle wriggling, squirming, and waving movements
- clenching and unclenching his fists
- opening his mouth and making "rooting" movements (see "Your Baby Knows How to Breastfeed," page 33)
- making sucking noises or smacking his lips
- murmuring, squeaking, whimpering, or giving little cries
- sucking his fists/clothes/blanket or your T-shirt/sweater

"Emily wasn't happy for the first month or two. In retrospect it's obvious I just wasn't feeding her enough. I'd nurse her and sometimes she'd want more twenty minutes later. I'd see all the signs but I didn't believe she needed it so I'd try to jiggle her to stop her crying. So she was miserable a lot of the time. I knew nursing would work but it felt like cheating—it was too easy."

Jane, mother of Emily, 5 years

ONE BREAST OR TWO?

Whether your baby feeds from one breast or both at each feeding is up to him and how hungry or thirsty he is. Just let him nurse for as long as he wants on the first breast and then, when he lets go, offer him the second. If he still seems hungry after that, try him on the first again.

It doesn't really matter which one he starts with each time, but feeding from the fuller one first will be best for your comfort. If your baby has a favorite breast, it's likely to make more milk and may be noticeably bigger than the other one in the early weeks, especially just before a feeding. The difference will soon become much less obvious, and once breastfeeding is over, both breasts will return to the same size.

What Else Your Baby Can Tell You

Breastfeeding is a skill you and your baby have to learn together. Part of trusting him to lead the way is recognizing his feeding cues and respecting his instinctive knowledge of what to do at the breast. But the other part is recognizing when he's trying to tell you that something is wrong.

Some babies who are finding breastfeeding difficult try to signal to their mother by squirming, pulling on and off the breast, and crying (they are often labeled "difficult feeders" or "breast refusers"). Others just resign themselves to the situation, becoming lethargic and reluctant to feed. Often, the problem isn't spotted until someone notices that the baby isn't gaining weight. If your instinct tells you something isn't right, ask for help (see "Where Can I Get Help?," page 108).

FEED BEFORE YOUR BREASTS GET TOO FULL

It can be tempting to make your baby wait until your breasts feel really full before letting him nurse, but this won't encourage him to take more milk or sleep longer between feedings; waiting is more likely to make him fussy and lead to him having difficulty latching on or coping with the milk flow. *Not* waiting until your breasts are overfull—or your baby is desperately hungry—before you let him feed is one of the secrets of effortless and relaxed breastfeeding.

Your Breasts in the First Two Weeks

Your breasts probably won't feel very different for a day or so after your baby is born, but there is a lot going on inside them: The blood supply is increasing and surges of prolactin are stimulating the milk-making cells into full-scale production. After a day or two, you may notice the thick, concentrated colostrum gradually changing, becoming more watery and less yellow, and your breasts may start to feel full.

Breast milk doesn't suddenly "come in" on the third day, and your breasts shouldn't be hard, swollen, shiny, or red, although they may be tender. "Third-day engorgement" is often thought of as normal just because most mothers experience it. However, it is actually the result of restricting breastfeeding and taking babies away from their mother (and giving them formula) at night.

Allowing your breasts to become overfull will not only be painful for you but will also make it difficult for your baby to latch on, so if you do start to feel uncomfortable, just offer your breast to your baby. If he seems to be struggling to attach, hand express a little milk (see page 87) to soften your breast and make it easier for him.

It can take a week or two for your let-down reflex (see page 22) to work in sync with your baby. Until then it's likely to happen randomly or to take a while to work when your baby is at your breast. Offering your baby the chance to nurse whenever you notice a tingling sensation or a sudden leakage of milk will help it begin to work more reliably. Once your body has learned what to do, you may find that the reflex is triggered just by thinking about feeding your baby, or by hearing him (or someone else's baby) cry.

In the first two weeks, your breasts will normally feel fuller before a feeding than they do afterward, but this will change as they start to respond more accurately to your baby's needs (see page 126). It's a good idea to get used to handling them so that you can detect any problems early (see "Painful Breastfeeding: Quick Symptom Checker," page 285).

What Can I Do About Leaking Milk?

Some women never leak milk, others leak often, and some leak more from one breast than from the other. It's particularly common to leak milk when the let-down reflex occurs, especially in the early weeks. (If your baby is nursing when this happens, you can expect the other breast to leak.)

If you know you're prone to leaking, you'll probably want to wear breast pads (commercial or homemade), so that you don't get damp patches on your clothes. Something thick and absorbent, which allows the skin to breathe, is better than something with a plastic backing, which may make a thrush infection (see page 240) more likely.

If you leak profusely from one breast while feeding from the other, you may find a milk collector (a hollow plastic device that you put inside your bra) more effective than a breast pad. If you make sure the milk collector is thoroughly clean beforehand, you'll be able to save the milk. It's not a good idea to wear a milk collector *between* feedings, since it tends to press into the breast—encouraging even more leakage—and it doesn't allow the skin to breathe.

TIPS FOR MANAGING UNEXPECTED LEAKS

- If you feel your let-down reflex starting to work at an inconvenient moment, pressing the heels of your hands against your breasts may be enough to stop it in its tracks. If you're in company you can probably do this discreetly, just by folding your arms or pressing your elbow against your breast. (You can fiddle with an earring, so it's not obvious.)
- Wearing a loose, patterned top rather than a tight, plain one will mean the occasional damp patch is less noticeable—or you may want to carry a cardigan or scarf so you can cover up easily.

If Your Milk Flows Too Rapidly for Your Baby

It's quite common for babies to struggle to cope with the flow of milk in the first few weeks, especially at the beginning of a feeding when the let-down reflex is at its strongest. Sometimes one breast has faster flow than the other. If your baby pulls away from the breast coughing and spluttering, there are several things you can do to help him:

- Take your baby off the breast for a few seconds when you feel the let-down reflex starting, then let him feed again once it's died down. If he seems uncomfortable, hold him upright for a few minutes so that he can bring up any air he may have swallowed.
- Express some milk before your baby begins feeding, to trigger the reflex. Wait until the flow subsides (or the tingling sensation stops) before offering him the breast.
- Hold your baby in a lying-back feeding position (as in photo 21), so that his head is higher than your breast (sometimes referred to as feeding "uphill"). This will lessen the force of the flow and make it easier for him to clear his airway if he does start to sputter. Sitting him upright, straddling your thigh, to feed can help, too (see photo 30).

SUCKING BLISTERS

Many babies develop sucking blisters—especially on their top lip—in the first week or so of breastfeeding, while they are getting the hang of it. The blisters don't seem to bother them and they don't need any treatment. They soon disappear.

Gas and Bringing Up Milk

Babies burp, pass gas, and bring up milk as a normal part of feeding, whether they are breastfed or formula fed. It can help to understand why this happens—and what, if anything, you need to do about it.

Do I Need to Burp My Baby?

Breastfed babies don't usually need burping after feedings. They may swallow small amounts of air as they feed, but this usually comes up by itself, as a burp. If your baby is settled and calm after a feeding (and particularly if he has fallen asleep while nursing), there is no need to disturb him by rubbing or banging him vigorously on the back. If he *does* have any gas, it isn't causing him a problem and he will get rid of it on his own.

Babies are more likely to swallow air while they're feeding if their attachment at the breast is ineffective or if the flow of milk is very fast. They also swallow air as they cry. If your baby is struggling to cope with a rush of milk or has had to wait to nurse, he may need the chance to bring up gas after the first few minutes. (See page 80 for tips on dealing with a rapid milk flow.) Just sitting him upright or holding him against your shoulder will usually be enough to help him burp. Overvigorous burping can make problems such as spit-up and reflux (see the following page) worse.

Like adults, babies also make gas in their gut while they're digesting their food (including breast milk). This gas can't be brought upward by burping—it has to go downward. Babies don't usually pass much more gas than do their parents, and it rarely causes them pain.

Is It Normal For Babies to Bring Up Milk?

Most babies bring up small amounts of milk from their stomach when they burp. Technically, this is called gastro-esophageal reflux (GER), but it's more commonly known as "spitting up." It's the same thing as when your own food repeats on you. Because a baby's esophagus (the tube that goes from the mouth to the stomach) is much shorter than an adult's, some of the milk comes out of the top rather than going back down again.

Spit-up can be a bit messy and inconvenient but it rarely worries babies (and regurgitated breast milk doesn't smell sour). It is usually a sign that they have had a particularly large feeding, or possibly that they've fed very fast. It's also more common when the baby has to gulp the milk, for example, if the flow is very fast (see page 80).

Just occasionally, what appears to be simply spit-up is actually something more serious, such as reflux disease or the projectile vomiting of pyloric stenosis (see boxes, below and on the following page). Both of these are more likely to be a problem if the baby is formula fed than if he is breastfed, partly because formula is digested less quickly than breast milk, and partly because formula feedings tend to be bigger and further apart, causing the stomach to become overstretched. Small, frequent feedings of breast milk are generally easier for all babies to manage.

WHAT IS REFLUX DISEASE?

Some babies regurgitate their stomach contents so often that the lining of their esophagus is damaged. This condition is called gastro-esophageal reflux disease (GERD). It can lead to pain (and crying) during and after feedings, as well as breathing difficulties, poor weight gain, and breast refusal. Some babies that are labeled as having colic in fact have GERD.

Thickeners (given before a breastfeeding) are sometimes recommended for babies with GERD. However, while these reduce the amount of milk the baby brings right up, they don't actually stop the regurgitation, so they don't prevent damage to the esophagus. There is a specific medicine that can help, but eventually babies outgrow the condition.

Pressure on the stomach, such as when a baby is sitting slumped in a car seat, makes spit-up more likely and can make the symptoms of reflux worse. For the first half an hour after nursing, your baby may be more comfortable in an upright position, with his legs dangling, than either propped up or lying down, and so a sling may be useful.

If you have any concerns about the amount of milk your baby is bringing up, discuss it with your doctor.

PROJECTILE VOMITING

Projectile vomiting can be a sign of pyloric stenosis, in which the muscle at the lower end of the stomach is unusually tight. If the stomach gets overfull, the contents get thrown back up forcefully. (Forceful vomiting can sometimes accompany a stomach infection, but in that case the baby will have other signs of illness.) If vomiting is severe and frequent, the baby may not be able to keep enough milk down to gain weight. Sometimes the condition can be treated with medication to relax the muscle, but it may require a small operation.

Newborn Jaundice—What's Normal and What Isn't

It's common for babies to develop mild jaundice on their second or third day because their liver isn't very efficient at filtering a substance called bilirubin (produced by the breakdown of excess red blood cells) from their blood. Jaundice causes the skin and the whites of the eyes to get a yellowy tinge, but it is not usually serious.

If the baby is feeding well, he will be pooping frequently, which gets rid of bilirubin, so the jaundice will disappear quickly (usually by the end of the first week). However, if he isn't taking much milk, some of the bilirubin will be reabsorbed from his gut and the jaundice will take longer to clear. Unfortunately, jaundiced babies tend to be sleepy, so they don't ask to nurse as often as they should (and they may not feed effectively). This can lead to a vicious cycle, in which the mother's breasts aren't given enough stimulation and milk production goes down—which means the baby gets even less milk and the jaundice gets worse.

If breastfeeding gets off to a good start, jaundice is unlikely to be a problem and feeding can be baby led. But if your baby is jaundiced and not nursing frequently—especially if he isn't producing many pees and poops (see page 99)—you will need to encourage him to nurse more often (see "If Your Baby Needs Encouragement to Feed," page 65). When he does attach, check that he is feeding effectively (see page 48—ask someone who knows about breastfeeding if you're unsure). Persuading him to take even small amounts of milk will give him more energy for nursing *and* help get rid of the jaundice; simply waiting for his appetite to improve won't do either.

Depending on the severity of the jaundice, your health-care provider may suggest ultraviolet light therapy (phototherapy) to help reduce it. Being under a warm light for long periods of time can make a baby dehydrated, so frequent breastfeeding is even more important.

Formula is sometimes suggested for jaundiced babies, to "flush their system through" and get rid of the bilirubin. This is unnecessary. Colostrum has a laxative effect, so it is just as good as formula at encouraging babies to poop frequently.

"Ella got jaundice and was put in an incubator. I was told to give her some formula because she needed lots of liquid. I gave her two formula feedings but I was so upset. After that I breastfed her every hour. I'd get her out of the incubator and hold her skin to skin with a blanket round us both and she'd feed. I think being a second-time mom I had the confidence to follow my instincts. She didn't need formula—she was fine and she's fed really well since then."

Sharon, mother of Daniel, 5 years,
and Ella, 7 weeks

So-called breast milk jaundice is much less common than newborn jaundice. It occurs only in breastfeeding babies and it doesn't usually appear until the baby is about two weeks old. The cause isn't fully understood, but some mothers find it happens in all their babies.

Unlike a baby with prolonged newborn jaundice, the baby with breast milk jaundice is alert, asking for feedings frequently, peeing and pooping normally, and gaining weight. So, although it can last for several weeks or even months, this type of jaundice doesn't usually need any treatment. However, it can overlap with newborn jaundice if the newborn type is slow to clear because of ineffective or infrequent feeding. If your baby hasn't had a period *without* jaundice, the first thing to check is that he's getting enough milk.

Occasionally, a baby will develop jaundice for another reason, such as an infection or a problem with his liver. If your doctor suspects that your baby's jaundice may be anything other than normal, he or she will order tests to find out what's wrong.

Learning to Hand Express Your Breast Milk

Expressing milk by hand is easy to do and can be useful in lots of ways. For example, in the early days, it can help relieve an overfull breast so that your baby can feed easily; later on, it can be used to clear a blocked duct (see page 245).

Hand expression tends to be better than a breast pump at triggering the release of hormones (helping milk production and flow) and it can be gentler, too. Some women find it quicker, even for expressing large amounts (e.g., for a premature baby, see page 193, or to leave with a babysitter, see Chapter 9), because there is no equipment to sterilize or assemble. You can do it whenever you need to and wherever you are; it costs nothing and you always have it—literally—at your fingertips.

The first two weeks are an ideal opportunity to practice hand expressing so that you have the knack when you need to use it. Sometimes mothers are advised *not* to express in the first six weeks. However, it's not the expressing that's the problem—it's giving expressed milk *by bottle* while a baby is learning to breastfeed (see "Breastfeeding Is Different from Bottle Feeding," page 32). You can express your milk as early as you like.

HOW TO EXPRESS YOUR MILK BY HAND, STEP BY STEP

Before you start, you may need to stimulate your let-down reflex to get your milk flowing, by thinking about your baby, holding him skin to skin, or *gently* massaging or stroking your breast. There's no need to massage or stroke in a particular way, just do whatever feels nice. Don't expect much milk the first time you express—it can take some practice. (The tips on page 152 will help if you want to express lots of milk.)

When you express your milk by hand, you are mimicking what your baby does with his mouth when he feeds (see page 31). Just like him, you need to find a spot a little way back from the nipple

(Continued on next page)

to squeeze the ducts so that the milk comes out. Here's how to do it:

1. Cup your breast in your (clean) hand with your thumb on top, in a C shape. (It's usually easiest to use the right hand on the right breast and the left hand on the left.)

2. Position your thumb and forefinger above and below your nipple, about one inch away from it.

3. Gently press your thumb and forefinger together. You should feel some breast tissue between them (it may feel gristly or lumpy). If all you feel is loose skin, try again, this time pressing backward into your breast before you squeeze. Experiment with moving your finger and thumb slightly farther back from the nipple until you find the right spot. There is normally no need to go farther back than your baby reaches with his mouth when he feeds.

4. Now squeeze slightly more firmly, to compress the ducts. Release, then squeeze again (without dragging your fingers across your skin). Build up a rhythm of press and release.

5. If you are squeezing in the right place, you'll begin to see drops of milk emerging. The first milk, colostrum, is quite sticky, but if your baby is more than a few days old, you may get fine jets or squirts (as in photo 5). If you don't see anything after a few squeezes, experiment with moving your thumb and finger closer to the nipple or farther away.

6. Once you know how far from your nipple your fingers need to be, pressing in different places around an imaginary circle will get milk from all parts of the breast. If you have a blocked duct or mastitis, placing your thumb on the red or lumpy side of the breast will target that area (see also Chapter 13).

If all you want to do is soften an overfull breast so your baby can attach, a few squeezes at two or three different spots on your imaginary circle will probably be enough. If you want to express lots of milk, just keep going in one position until the flow subsides before moving to the next.

If you don't need to save the milk, you can express into any container or just over the sink. If you do want to keep the milk, use a thoroughly clean bowl or large cup to catch it. (Breast milk often squirts in different directions, so choose a wide-mouthed one.) If you are expressing for a preterm or sick baby, make sure the container you use is sterilized beforehand. See page 154 for information on storing breast milk.

From Now on It Gets Easier

The first two weeks of breastfeeding can be pretty busy and at times it will feel as though you're doing nothing but breastfeeding. But once this time is over, both you and your baby will be getting familiar with the practicalities of nursing and learning to trust each other. From now on his feedings will still need to be **Frequent**, **Effective**, **Exclusive**, and on **Demand** (see page 71)—and **Skin** to skin, when you get the chance—but, as you and he get more in tune with each other and your confidence grows, you'll find yourself nursing him without even thinking about it.

It may not feel like a huge milestone, but by focusing on breast-feeding for these two weeks, you have set up your long-term capacity to produce as much milk as your baby needs and laid the foundations for an easy and rewarding breastfeeding relationship.

KEY POINTS

- Having a two-week babymoon after your baby is born can make concentrating on breastfeeding easier. Accept help with your other responsibilities.
- Try not to share your baby too much during this time— you can easily miss feeding cues if someone else is holding him.
- Encourage your baby to nurse frequently in the first couple of weeks, to set your breasts up for maximum milk production, help you avoid engorgement, and give you both plenty of practice.
- Hold your baby skin to skin whenever you can and keep him near you day and night.
- Avoid giving your baby formula or water unless there are medical reasons why he needs them—at least for the first two weeks but preferably for the first six months.
- Avoid giving your baby a pacifier or feeding him with a bottle—at least for the first two weeks.
- Get to know your breasts and how they feel now they're "working."
- Learn to express your milk by hand.

6

Knowing It's Working

"THE PROBLEM WITH breastfeeding is that you can't see how much the baby is getting." This is a familiar lament. Many women worry about whether their baby is having enough milk, especially in the early weeks. Breastfeeding babies regulate their own appetites, so the only person who really knows whether she's getting enough milk is your baby. Part of baby-led breastfeeding involves learning to recognize the everyday signs that will tell you how well nursing is going—from your point of view and your baby's. This chapter shows you how.

Knowing What to Look For

For many decades most people in the United States—including health professionals—have been more familiar with formula feeding than with breastfeeding. The behavior of formula-fed babies (regular feedings with long periods of sleep), together with their average intake of milk (which can be measured exactly), have been used as benchmarks for judging whether a baby is getting enough.

The parent-led nature of formula feeding has made us wary of trusting babies to decide for themselves how often to feed and how long to feed for—especially when we can't see how much milk they're taking. So when a baby has an erratic pattern, with frequent feedings of varying lengths (perfectly normal for a breastfed baby), it's easy to assume that something is wrong.

> "I was confused by the irregularity of Kyla's feedings in the early weeks—especially when she wanted to nurse all the time in the evening. I was convinced feedings should be evenly spaced and I'd get really worried that she didn't have a pattern. But she did—it just wasn't the one I thought she should have."
>
> Eva, mother of Kyla, 7 months

Breastfed babies naturally feed at different speeds, so watching the clock won't tell you how much milk your baby is taking. In general, babies get faster at nursing as they mature, but even then, the same baby can choose to take her time during some feedings and race through others (even if she takes the same amount of milk each time)—just as you do with your meals. Breast milk also varies among mothers and throughout the day (see page 27). All of this means that it's impossible to measure how much milk your baby is taking—or even to know exactly how much she needs. But you don't need to: Your baby is the one who makes these decisions. What you *can* do is figure out if what she's getting is enough to keep her healthy and help her grow—and there are lots of signs you can look for:

- Watching and listening to your baby while she's feeding will tell you whether she's taking plenty of milk at *this* feeding.
- How your breasts feel and look immediately after a feeding will tell you what happened during that feeding (as well as helping you spot signs of infection or other problems).

- Your baby's pees and poops will tell you what's been happening over the last few hours.
- Your baby's behavior, weight, and general appearance will tell you what's been happening over the last few days.

Watching and Listening to Your Baby Feed

Breastfed babies have a typical pattern of sucking and swallowing during feedings. How well your baby fits this pattern each time she nurses—and how she ends the feeding—will reveal a lot about whether she's getting lots of milk.

What Happens at the Beginning of the Feeding

Most babies will attach to the breast fairly quickly as long as they are calm, ready to feed, and can scoop up a good mouthful easily. Some babies come on and off the breast several times before they start to suck as they work to get the nipple into the most comfortable place. Unless your baby is lying on top of you (in which case she can adjust her position herself), you may need to be ready to modify the way you're holding her, to make it easier for her to get the right angle.

A baby who persistently attaches and lets go at the start of a feeding *may* have a tongue tie (see page 38) that is making it difficult for her to attach effectively. If she comes off the breast crying after a few sucks or doesn't seem to want to go near it at all, the problem could be "breast refusal," which has many possible causes (see "If Your Baby Goes on Strike," page 129). Remember that a baby who has had to wait to nurse and has been crying may simply be finding it difficult to calm down enough to latch on—or she may have a tummy full of gas (see page 81).

Watching and Listening for Sucking and Swallowing

It's a good idea to spend some time in the first week getting to know your baby's pattern of sucking and swallowing. During the first couple of days, while she is having mainly colostrum, she may not swallow very often. However, from the third day onward you should be able to see (or hear) her sucking and swallowing in this sort of pattern:

- At the beginning of the feeding, there will probably be a burst of short, rapid sucks with little or no swallowing. This could last a second or two or it could last a few minutes. During this time, your baby is making sure she has your nipple a long way back in her mouth and is waiting for your let-down reflex to work.
- Once your milk is flowing, as long as she is effectively attached, your baby will relax and settle down to a pattern of big yawning sucks (see page 31) and swallows—usually one or two "yawns" to each swallow. This rhythm tells you that she is getting a big mouthful of milk with each suck. Some babies swallow very loudly; some make a little "cuh" sound, and others swallow almost silently, with just a little outward breath (like a quick puff of air) from their nose after each one. Sometimes it's easier to see a baby swallow than to hear her. If your baby is swallowing, she's getting milk.
- If your baby wants just a small drink, she will stop feeding quite quickly. If not, she'll carry on in short bursts of "yawns" and swallows, with occasional pauses for a rest.
- After a while, as the milk gets gradually thicker and creamier (see page 27), the flow will start to slow down and you'll notice her swallowing less frequently.
- As your baby gets ready to come off the breast, her pauses will get longer and she'll do very little swallowing. She may look as

though she is falling asleep. Her chin may quiver slightly, followed by a short flurry of quick sucks (called "flutter sucking"), and another long pause. It's tempting to assume, if you notice this, that she is just sucking for comfort and that you should take her off the breast, but this is when your milk is at its creamiest. She's still getting food—in small amounts but packed full of calories. She will come off by herself—but not quite yet.

- When she lets go, she may want to continue feeding on your other breast, either right away or after a rest, taking just a few sucks or going through the whole cycle again, depending on her hunger.

This pattern is very different from that of a baby feeding from a bottle, whose suck-swallow rhythm stays more or less the same throughout. Bottle feeding is more tiring for babies because they have to pause frequently to take a breath, whereas a breastfeeding baby can breathe while she sucks.

WHAT'S THAT CLICKING NOISE?

Some babies make a loud "clicking" noise when they feed. (This usually occurs when the jaw is at its widest and shouldn't be confused with the audible "glug" that can accompany swallowing.) Clicking indicates a loss of suction, and it can be a sign of an unusually high palate or a tongue tie. If feeding is otherwise going well, you can ignore the clicking. However, if your baby always takes a long time to nurse, seems exhausted by sucking, or is not producing the expected number of pees and poops—or if you are experiencing pain when nursing—then it may be significant. In that case, improving your baby's attachment may be all that's needed, but if the clicking doesn't stop, seek expert help.

Your Baby Will End the Feeding

Babies *always* come off the breast by themselves when they've had enough milk. If they don't, they haven't. Typically, the baby's sucking will slow down as she reaches the creamiest milk near the end of the feeding (see page 27), until eventually she pushes the nipple out with her tongue. She may smack her lips and have a satisfied "drunk" look on her face—like the baby in photo 7.

Babies often fall asleep at the breast. This is the most natural thing in the world, but it can occasionally be a sign that breastfeeding is not going well. A baby who is ineffectively attached has to work hard to get milk and may fall asleep because she's exhausted. Unlike the baby who's had enough milk (who will usually stay asleep), she'll often wake up as the nipple falls out of her mouth and want to go right back on again, because she didn't mean to let go and her tummy isn't full.

A breastfeeding can be as short as a few sucks or as long as three quarters of an hour. And a baby can feed from just one breast or both— or even go from one to the other several times. Only your baby knows what she needs at that particular feeding and only she knows when she's had it. But if she consistently wants to nurse for longer than about forty-five minutes, or falls asleep at the breast and is awake again (and asking to feed) ten minutes later, it's worth checking her attachment.

USING BREASTFEEDING TO SETTLE YOUR BABY

For a baby, breastfeeding is comforting and soothing—a lovely way to drift off to sleep. Allowing your baby to relax and let go of the breast in her own time is a good thing, not a bad one. She will gradually find ways to settle herself and fall asleep on her own, but she doesn't need to be deprived of her main source of comfort in order to do that.

If It Hurts, It's Not Right

Painful breastfeeding—even in the first few weeks—is a sign that something is wrong. And even if your baby *seems* to be feeding well, if it's hurting you, it's probably not right for her, either.

Your nipples may be slightly sensitive in the first few days—a few seconds of "ouch" at the beginning of a feeding isn't unusual (see page 36). But that's all. After that, the feeding should be pain free. Mostly, the reason for painful breastfeeding is that the baby isn't attached effectively, which means she won't be getting as much milk as she should. Occasionally, it's caused by an infection. Either way, it needs attention quickly, so if you can't fix it yourself (see "Painful Breastfeeding: Quick Symptom Checker," page 285), you will need to get some help.

When your baby comes off your breast, it's a good idea to check that your nipple is the same shape and color as it was before it went in. It may look a bit longer, because it's been slightly stretched, but it shouldn't look pinched or wedge-shaped, or be white or blue (see page 236). If it *is* an odd shape or color, it's probably been squashed against the hard part of the roof of her mouth or between her gums, because she hasn't taken in a big enough mouthful of breast.

Feeling your breasts for lumps and bumps occasionally (maybe once a day, after nursing) is a good way to make sure you pick up problems such as blocked ducts early, so you can deal with them before they become painful. See "Painful Breastfeeding: Quick Symptom Checker," page 285, for what to do if you find something unusual.

SIGNS THAT YOUR BABY IS FEEDING EFFECTIVELY

- Her body is relaxed, not tense, while she's feeding.
- She feeds rhythmically, with slow, deep sucks and occasional pauses.
- She swallows after every one or two sucks for most of the feeding.
- The pauses get gradually longer and the swallows less frequent.
- She pushes or spits your nipple out of her mouth and looks satisfied.
- Your nipples are the same shape and color after the feeding as they were before.
- Nursing doesn't hurt and your nipples and breasts aren't sore.

SIGNS THAT NEED ATTENTION

- Your baby comes on and off the breast during a feeding.
- Her sucking is shallow and erratic rather than deep and rhythmic.
- She swallows only after every three or more sucks.
- She never takes herself off the breast, or she falls off and then wants to feed again immediately.
- One or both of your nipples is an odd shape or color when it comes out of your baby's mouth.
- One or both of your nipples hurts all the time your baby is feeding, or is cracked or bleeding.
- Your breasts are sore, painful, lumpy, or inflamed.

What You Can See by Your Baby's Pee (and Why Her Poop Is Worth a Snoop)

One of the best ways to tell whether your baby is getting enough milk is to check her pees and poops. If there's enough going in, there will be plenty coming out.

Pees are the best guide to how much milk your baby has had in the last six to twelve hours. Poops (together with pees) are the best guide to how much milk your baby has had in the last twenty-four hours. (This assumes she is having only your milk. If she is being given anything else—even water—her pees and poops won't give a reliable picture.)

> "I had no confidence when I came home from hospital. I was convinced I didn't have enough milk. Olivia wanted to be on the breast all the time so I thought she must be starving. I made notes of all her feedings to show her doctor. Eventually I realized it was normal for her to nurse that much and that I could easily tell by her diapers that she was getting enough milk."
>
> Kate, mother of Olivia, 5 months

How Often Should My Baby Pee?

Babies don't need to drink much for the first few days and the early milk (colostrum) is very concentrated, so breastfed babies don't pass much urine during this time. If you were given a lot of IV fluids in labor you may find your baby pees a lot the first day, but in general a good guide for the first five days is to expect *at least* one pee on the first day, two on the second, three on the third, and so on. After this, your baby should be producing at least six pale yellow pees every day. If her milk intake suddenly goes up or down, you will notice a change in her pees within a few hours.

Urine doesn't show up very well in some diapers (especially the disposable type), so the best guide is how heavy the diaper is. Pouring an ounce and a half (three tablespoons) of water into a dry diaper will give you an idea of how it should feel.

PINK PEE

Sometimes the diaper of a newborn baby contains pinkish or orangey spots. These are urate crystals, which occasionally form in concentrated urine. This is quite normal and doesn't usually last more than a day or two because, as milk production gets going, the baby is drinking more.

What Should My Baby's Poops Look Like?

Changes in your baby's poop in the first five days will show you how well she is feeding. The first stool is meconium, which is very thick, sticky, and black or greenish-black in color. You can expect your baby to pass meconium two or three times before the color starts to change. (Some babies pass meconium during labor as well.)

Sometime between twenty-four and forty-eight hours after the birth you will probably notice the poop becoming slightly less sticky and more yellowish-green in color. This is known as a "transition stool," and it's a sign that milk has begun to work its way through your baby's digestive system. It will then get progressively more orangey-yellow in color and more runny, until, by day four or five, it's like runny yellow mustard. Photos 8 to 10 show what you can expect your baby's poop to look like over the first five days.

The amount of poop is more variable than that of pees, but from her second day onward, your baby should be producing *at least* two teaspoonful-size poops (or larger) per day. If she isn't producing runny yellow poops by her fifth day, it's likely that she hasn't been getting all the milk she should. In that case, ask for someone to check her feeding technique and suggest some adjustments (see "Where Can I Get Help?," page 108).

PEES AND POOPS IN THE FIRST FIVE DAYS

DAY AFTER BIRTH	PEE		POOP	
	Appearance	How many times in 24 hours?	Appearance	How many times in 24 hours?
1st	Pale yellow; may contain pinkish spots	At least 1	Thick, sticky, greenish-black	At least 1
2nd	Pale yellow	At least 2	Less sticky; more yellowish-green ("transition stool")	At least 2
3rd	Pale yellow	At least 3	Runnier and more yellow	At least 2; probably 3 or more
4th	Pale yellow	At least 4	Runnier and more orangey-yellow	At least 2; probably 4 or more
5th	Pale yellow	At least 5	Runny; orangey-yellow (like yellow mustard)	At least 2; probably 5 or more
After this	Pale yellow	At least 6	Runny; orangey-yellow (like yellow mustard)	At least 2; probably 6 or more (until at least 4 weeks)

Your baby should continue to produce at least two poops (and probably more) per day for the first four to six weeks. After this, her stools may suddenly become less frequent and she may go for several days (maybe even a week or more) without producing a poop at all. This is quite normal—but *not* in the first few weeks. If it happens then, it suggests she isn't taking in enough milk.

The color of your baby's poop may vary a bit between orange and green, but mostly it will stay yellow (and runny) all the time she is on breast milk alone. It may appear to have "seeds" in it sometimes; this is normal. People who are used to the darker, more solid poop of a formula-fed baby sometimes think that breast milk must be "going straight through," or that the baby has diarrhea. But it's this yellow, runny, slightly sweet-smelling type of poop that babies are supposed to produce. (See "What to Expect When" on page 280 for a quick summary.)

> "I couldn't believe how much poop Ethan produced. After a few weeks, he stopped going so often—he just used to save it up and then there'd be a massive explosion—up to his neck and down to his knees! At least it didn't smell bad."
>
> Chantelle, mother of Ethan, 10 months

Your Baby's Behavior Can Tell You a Lot

Your baby's nursing pattern will be unique and no two days will be exactly the same. But how she behaves between feedings and when she comes to the breast can tell you a lot about how breastfeeding is going.

The Too-Contented Baby

Most babies who aren't getting enough milk let their parents know, by asking vigorously for feedings and crying a lot. But some babies don't have enough energy to do this, either because they haven't been getting much milk for quite a while, because they are premature (see Chapter 11), or because they are sick. They may show only fleeting feeding cues and sleep most of the time—and the fact that something is wrong can easily go unnoticed.

Babies are not supposed to feed infrequently and sleep for long periods. They should have periods of alertness, when they are looking around and wanting to be talked to. And they should want to feed often. If your baby is asking to nurse fewer than six times in twenty-four hours (eight times every twenty-four hours in the first two weeks) and sleeping almost all the time—especially if she is jaundiced (see page 84)—look carefully at her behavior during feedings and check her pees and poops. If in doubt, seek help (see "Where Can I Get Help?," page 108).

Expecting a baby to feed infrequently and to spend much of the day on her own or sleeping (often referred to as being "contented") is not realistic or safe—and it's not good for breastfeeding.

The "Colicky" Baby

Babies who cry a lot are often said to have "colic." It tends to be more common in the evenings and is thought by many people to indicate tummy-ache. However, it's not always clear that the problem really *is* tummy-ache. Many colicky babies settle down if they are held or offered a feeding, suggesting that they were just hungry or needing extra reassurance. Some babies who are diagnosed with "evening colic" simply need to nurse a lot in the evenings (see "Babies Like to Feed in Clusters," page 114); not responding to them when they ask makes them upset. And babies who have to wait to be fed can be colicky because they've swallowed air while crying. However, if your baby is colicky and none of the above scenarios applies, the problem could be "breastfeeding colic."

A baby who has breastfeeding colic usually cries (or screams) for long periods soon after a feeding. She is difficult to console, often drawing her knees up toward her chest or arching her back. Her poop is likely to be quite distinctive—greenish, watery-looking, maybe even frothy—and there's lots of it.

Babies with breastfeeding colic tend to want to feed very frequently and some don't gain weight as they should. Because of this, mothers whose baby is colicky are sometimes told that their milk isn't rich enough for their baby, or that it doesn't suit her. This isn't true—there's nothing wrong with the milk. The answer lies in the feeding.

There are two main reasons for breastfeeding colic:

- The baby is not feeding effectively.
- The baby is not able to feed for long enough.

Either of these will mean your baby will tend to get the watery—and sugary—"soup course" but she won't get as far as the creamy, fat-laden "dessert," which is an essential part of the feeding. So she ends up with too much sugar compared with the amount of fat. This causes the milk to rush through the gut without being fully digested, giving the poop its green color and watery consistency. The excess sugar ferments, producing gas, which causes pain. The combination of an irritated gut and lots of gas results in "explosive" stools that are passed fast and noisily and a baby who is miserable.

If your baby has the symptoms of breastfeeding colic, have a careful look at the way she is feeding. Make sure she gets a good mouthful of breast (see page 30), and let her nurse for as long as she wants. This will mean she'll get all the fat she should. You'll probably notice a difference in her behavior and her poop within twenty-four hours—possibly sooner. In the meantime, holding her in an upright position or giving her a gentle massage or some skin-to-skin time may help make her more comfortable.

A less common cause of colic occurring after the first few weeks is that the mother is producing excessive amounts of milk, so her baby gets too much of the thinner milk and has no room for the creamier milk (see "Could I Be Making Too Much Milk?," page 219). Occasionally it can be the result of something the mother has eaten (see page 135). Rarely, colicky behavior is a sign of a more serious condition, such as reflux disease (see page 83). If you can't identify the cause of your baby's crying, ask your doctor to check her over.

> "My grandma and my friends were pressuring me to bottle feed because Tom was so colicky—they kept saying I didn't have enough milk. But I just *knew* he wasn't hungry. Eventually I saw a breastfeeding supporter and she explained I'd been taking him off the breast too soon. I thought he'd fallen asleep when he was still going. Once I stopped doing that he was fine—and much happier."
>
> Becky, mother of Tom, 9 months

If Your Baby Refuses to Feed

Having your baby refuse the breast, cry loudly, and arch her back to avoid it can be distressing for both of you. While your nurturing instinct is telling you to hold her close, she seems to be pushing you away.

The most common cause of breast refusal in a young baby is that the baby has been repeatedly held in an uncomfortable or awkward position for nursing. This makes breastfeeding unpleasant and frustrating for her, and she will associate the breast with these feelings. It's very difficult for a baby to breastfeed if she can't tilt her head back or if she has to twist her head sideways to get to the breast. She'll struggle to open her mouth wide enough to feed and it will be difficult for her to swallow.

If you think your baby's position could be the problem, try adjusting the way you hold her so that she can feed more easily. Lying back with her on your tummy (see page 41) will allow her to feed with the minimum of handling and may help you both to get your confidence back. If this doesn't solve the problem, it may be that you need to concentrate on helping her feel happy near your breast again and get back to her instincts for breastfeeding. The way to do this is described on page 130.

Occasionally babies refuse the breast if it tastes or smells strange to them. This can happen when the mother uses scented wipes or soap on her nipples before feeding. There's no need to clean your nipples before you feed your baby.

If your baby is happy to feed for a minute or two and *then* pulls away, it could be that the milk flow is too fast for her, especially if she comes off spluttering. This is most likely to happen at the beginning of the feeding, when the let-down reflex is strongest. See page 80 for how to deal with this. Rarely, breast refusal is a sign of reflux disease (see page 83).

Occasionally, feeding is painful for a newborn baby because her skull bones are slightly out of alignment following the birth. Some parents have found that cranial osteopathy, craniosacral therapy, or chiropractic, in which the skull is gently manipulated back into shape, is helpful in these circumstances. If you can't find an obvious answer for your baby's refusal to feed, you may want to seek out a practitioner who specializes in cranial work and who is used to treating babies (see "Sources of Information and Support," page 292).

In a baby older than one month, a sudden episode of breast refusal (also called a "nursing strike") is more likely to be caused by something unconnected with the feeding itself. See page 129 for some possible causes, and for tips on what to do.

What to Expect with Your Baby's Weight

Many parents and health professionals put a lot of emphasis on a baby's weight; and as they grow, many babies are weighed much more often than they need to be. Weight *is* important, but it's not enough on its own to tell you whether breastfeeding is going well—and it's a fairly slow way of spotting feeding problems.

Weight Gain in the Early Days

It's normal for babies to lose a small amount of weight in the first few days. However, they shouldn't lose very much, and they will usually begin to gain weight again on about their fourth day, as milk production gets going. Excessive weight loss—10 percent or more—in the first few days can be a sign of illness, but more often it's an indication that the baby hasn't been getting enough milk.

Your baby's weight gain is related to how much milk she takes in. If she doesn't get the milk you are making, she won't thrive—and your breasts will start to cut down production (see "Production on Demand—How It Works," page 23). However, weight gain (or loss) doesn't tell you what's happening *now* with your baby's feedings, only what has happened over the past few days. Your baby's nursing behavior, and her pees and poops, are a much more immediate guide (see pages 99 and 102). If you ignore these signs and wait to see how much weight she has gained, your milk production may slow down in the meantime, giving you a double problem (still solvable, but not quite as easily).

If your baby is healthy, feeding effectively, and peeing and pooping normally, then (except in the first couple of days) she *will* be gaining weight. If her feeding technique, pees, and poops are all okay and she *isn't* gaining weight, then something else is wrong and she should be checked out by a doctor.

How Often Should I Weigh My Baby?

Babies tend to gain weight in an irregular pattern, rather than constantly. While she shouldn't *lose* weight after the first few days, or stay the same weight for very long at a time, there is no reason to expect your baby to put on weight at a steady rate, week after week, so there's no advantage in weighing her frequently. A couple of weight checks in the first two weeks is a good idea, just to make sure she is adjusting well to life outside the womb. After that, unless there are particular concerns about her health, there's no need to weigh her more than once a month. Every two months is fine after she reaches six months, and if you want to carry on having her weighed once she reaches a year, every three to six months is plenty.

What If It's Not Working?

When breastfeeding goes wrong, there's almost always a solution. The answer usually lies in going back to the basics. If you suspect that breastfeeding isn't going well, for either you or for your baby, start by looking at her feeding pattern over a twenty-four-hour period and watching her closely while she's feeding. A quiet day or two with plenty of skin-to-skin contact may be enough to put things right. Have another look at Chapters 3 and 5 to remind you what to look for and how to make sure feeding is effective. You may also find the information on starting breastfeeding late useful (see page 224). If you can't find the answer—or are struggling to change things—get some help.

Where Can I Get Help?

Your midwife or doctor may seem the most obvious person to turn to when you are concerned about your baby's feeding, but not all health professionals have had in-depth training on breastfeed-ing, so they may not necessarily be the best people to help. Some ob-gyn practices and hospitals offer breastfeeding classes, but one-on-one care is more usually provided by lactation consultants. Help is also available from volunteer breastfeeding counselors and support groups, some of which have telephone helplines. There are numerous websites, too, which provide breastfeeding information. See "Sources of Information and Support," page 289, for a few useful addresses.

KEY POINTS

- Watching and listening to your baby as she nurses will tell you whether she's getting milk. Look for a rhythm of big yawning sucks with frequent swallows that gradually slows down as the milk gets creamier.
- If your baby goes on and off the breast at the start of the feeding, she's probably finding it difficult to attach.
- If your baby doesn't come off the breast by herself, or if she almost always nurses for more than 45 minutes, check her attachment.
- Checking your nipples for damage after feedings, and your breasts for lumps and inflammation once a day, will help you spot breastfeeding problems early.
- Pees and poops are the best clues to whether your baby is getting enough milk.
- Babies under four weeks should poop at *least* twice a day; older babies may go several days without a poop.
- If your baby is miserable, feeds very frequently, and has green poop, check the way she's feeding.
- If a young baby refuses the breast, the most likely reason is that she is being held awkwardly.

- If your baby is sleepy and not asking for many feedings, seek help.
- Weight isn't the best way to check how breastfeeding is going—other signs (such as pees and poops) are more helpful.
- If you have any doubts about how breastfeeding is going, seek help. The earlier you find out what's wrong, the easier it will be to fix it.

7

Settling In to Breastfeeding

AS YOU FOLLOW your baby's lead, the intensity of the first few weeks of breastfeeding will gradually lessen. Your baby will develop a more predictable rhythm, and as you both gain experience, you'll start to feel that you don't need to concentrate so much each time he breastfeeds. This chapter is about the changes you can expect over the next few months, how to adjust to your baby's natural nursing pattern, and why trying to get him into a routine is unlikely to work. (For an overview of what to expect throughout the time your baby is breastfeeding, see "What to Expect When," page 280.)

Getting Breastfeeding "Established"

Technically, it takes about six weeks for milk production to become established—that is, for a mother's breasts to settle into a pattern of milk production that suits her baby. But after two or three weeks, you'll probably notice that your breasts feel less full between feedings, they leak less often, and your let-down reflex is more reliable.

Establishing *breastfeeding* is slightly different. It's about you and your baby learning to work together so that nursing is second nature, instead of something you have to concentrate on. It's about reaching the stage when you don't notice how many times your baby feeds over the course of the day and through the night, as you and he respond more intuitively to each other and breastfeeding requires less effort.

How long it will take for you and your baby to reach this level of confidence is difficult to predict. Even if you've breastfed a baby before, this new relationship will be different. Some mothers and babies are confident after a week or two; others can take a couple of months. You probably won't know until you look back and realize things suddenly feel much easier. The key is to give yourself and your baby plenty of time and opportunities to practice, and to trust each other.

Why Routines Don't Work

Attempting to impose your own schedule—or one from a book—is likely to disrupt breastfeeding. Most adult-designed routines are based on set times for nursing and sleeping (and sometimes even for playing). Usually there are quite long gaps between feedings. Breastfeeding isn't designed to work like this.

Breastfeeding is more than food and drink—it also provides babies with comfort, company, warmth, and security. None of these things can be regulated by the clock, so expecting your baby to fit into a schedule is unrealistic. For a mother, in the short term controlling or restricting nursing is likely to lead to engorgement (see page 243); in the longer term, it will cause less milk to be made. If you are one of the rare women who naturally overproduce milk, it's possible such a routine will work for *you*—but it probably won't work for your baby.

It's unlikely babies have any concept of the future. Their survival instincts tell them their need is urgent, and research suggests that if they don't get a quick response, they feel frightened.

Trying to fight your baby's instincts to nurse and be held will make him—and you—stressed and miserable. Responding to his needs promptly will make life easier for both of you. It's not about allowing your baby to rule your life; it's about adjusting your life to include your baby.

Your baby will eventually eat and sleep at conventional times, but not yet. In the meantime, making an active decision to let him lead the way will make breastfeeding—and parenting—much easier than trying to force things into a routine. Many families who start out trying to establish a routine quickly discover that keeping their baby near and responding to his needs is better for breastfeeding—and for family life generally.

> "The unpredictability of everything made me panicky in the first few months, so I started following a routine from a book, with three-hourly feedings, times to sleep, play, and have 'me-time.' I thought the structure would make me feel better but I ended up pacing around with Emily screaming, waiting for the three hours to be up. Even if I wanted a routine, it wasn't working for her—she was miserable. Eventually I realized a happy baby meant a happy mom. It had to be that way round—because no one is happy if the baby is screaming."
>
> Julie, mother of Emily, 18 months

Your Baby's Changing Patterns

For the first few weeks, your baby's feedings will probably be unpredictable, and life may feel quite chaotic. After that, although no two days will be exactly the same, you'll start to see a pattern emerging. He may start to nurse slightly less often at night, especially if he is able to feed frequently in the evenings. During the day, his appetite will vary (like yours), with some feedings very short and some quite long. He'll almost certainly continue to want to nurse at least six times in twenty-four hours—and probably many more—though it's unlikely you'll feel the need to count them.

> "I thought I was feeding on demand until I went to a baby group and I saw a woman *really* feeding on demand. I had no idea how she knew her baby needed to nurse but she'd be chatting away to someone and every now and then, almost without looking, she'd just lift him to her breast and he'd have a little feeding. She seemed completely in tune with him."
>
> Kim, mother of Sadie, 6 months

Babies Like to Feed in Clusters

Many babies want lots of feedings close together, in "clusters," especially in the evenings. (This is also known as bunch feeding.) They can get very distressed if their need to nurse isn't met, and this unsettled behavior and crying is often mistaken for colic (see page 103).

The constant on-off nature of cluster feeding can make ordinary tasks such as cooking a meal or cleaning up difficult. Getting to know your baby's individual pattern will make it easier for you to plan for this (for example, by preparing some of the meal in advance, using a slow cooker, or sharing the cooking with your partner).

Figuring out how to feed your baby in a sling can also help with cluster feeding, because it allows you to have your hands free to get on with other things, even if your baby is on and off the breast all evening. If there's nothing else you need to be doing, lying back on the couch with your baby on top of you, so he can latch on whenever he needs to, may be the easiest solution. That way *he* won't have to keep asking and *you* won't have to keep picking him up and rearranging your clothes.

Many (though not all) babies who develop a pattern of evening cluster feeding have a longer period of sleep afterward. Resisting your baby's requests for feeding is likely to make him unsettled all evening—and most of the night as well—whereas if you give in to what's happening and let him nurse on and off throughout the evening, you're likely to get more sleep.

"I wasted a lot of time and energy trying to fit my first baby's feedings into a pattern that worked for me but not for him. Once I resigned myself to sitting on the couch all evening and stopped trying to put my boobs away, it all seemed to get easier. I didn't make the same mistake with the next two when they wanted to feed all evening. I just read a book or watched TV while they nursed."

Margaret, mother of Paul, 10 years,
James, 9 years, and Lisa, 7 years

YOU DON'T ALWAYS HAVE TO WAIT FOR YOUR BABY TO ASK

Breastfeeding your baby whenever he wants may make you wonder whether you'll ever be able to plan anything. But you don't have to wait for him to ask every time. Most young babies are open to nursing whenever they're awake—and sometimes even when they're not! If you need to go out somewhere—or start a long journey—and don't want to risk your baby wanting to nurse the minute you set foot outside the door, you can offer him the opportunity to feed *before* he asks. If he's asleep, just rubbing his nose gently against your nipple or expressing a few drops of milk on to his lips may be enough to tempt him to at least have a quick snack.

Expect Appetite Spurts

Sometimes a baby will suddenly start to feed more frequently than usual and then settle back to a familiar nursing pattern after a few days. This is called an appetite spurt (or a growth spurt or hunger spurt). It happens because the baby is feeling extra hungry and needs to stimulate more milk (although it doesn't necessarily coincide with his growing faster than usual). A few days of increased nursing is all that's needed to give the breasts the message that they need to make more.

Feeding at Night

Nursing at night is important. Babies aren't born knowing that their parents have designated nighttime as sleep time. Most babies nurse more frequently in the evening and early part of the night (7:00 PM–3:00 AM) than they do in the early morning and during the day (3:00 AM–7:00 PM), for at least the first few weeks. Nursing as often as your baby needs, night and day, is the best way to ensure you make plenty of milk and avoid engorgement (see page 243). For breastfeeding to work well, you and your baby need to be in sync twenty-four hours a day.

> "It took me a long time to respond to Lilly instinctively during the day. There were so many distractions and I was a bit stressed. It was different at night. It's a different kind of sleep with a baby. I'd be asleep but also very aware of her movements, and I'd always wake up to nurse just before she stirred. I was much more in tune with her—it felt more instinctive and intimate."
>
> Hannah, mother of Lilly, 10 months

Pressure to get a baby to sleep all night can often come from people who think babies should be "taught" to manage on their own or who are used to formula feeding, which tends to be less frequent. But human babies aren't supposed to sleep too deeply; they're meant to wake frequently to feed. Nursing at night is easier if you don't *expect* your baby to sleep right through.

> "My mom was always asking if Nathan was sleeping through yet. So we just decided 'night' meant midnight to five am. That way we could tell her that Nathan only woke once! It took a bit of the pressure off."
>
> Kieran, father of Nathan, 3 months

Here are some tips for making breastfeeding at night easier to manage:

- Go to bed early if you can.
- Offer your baby a breastfeeding immediately before you go to bed. There's no need to wake him—just hold him next to your breast and talk to him gently, or express some milk onto his lips to encourage him to latch on.
- Keep your baby in the same room with you—or, provided it's safe (see box), in your bed. This will help coordinate your sleep cycle with his, so that you're already waking up when he starts to stir and can nurse him without either of you needing to wake up fully. (An alternative to bed sharing is a three-sided "arm's reach" or "co-sleeper" crib that clips on to your bed, allowing you to reach your baby easily.)
- Offer your baby a feeding as soon as he begins to wake, before he starts to cry.
- Learn to feed lying down, so you can rest while your baby feeds.

- Sleep naked, or wear an easy-to-open nightgown, pajama top, or bra. (If you tend to leak milk, spread a thick towel underneath your top half to protect the bed.)
- Learn to breastfeed in the dark so you don't have to wake everybody up by switching on the light (and so your baby doesn't start to associate darkness with being hungry or lonely and light with food and comfort). Practice during the day by feeding with your eyes shut.
- Don't change your baby's diaper at night unless it's very wet, he pooped, or he has a diaper rash.
- Have a drink nearby in case you are thirsty (so you don't have to get out of bed).
- Help your baby decide to do more of his feeding during the day by making a point of not tip-toeing around him in the mornings—even if you're grateful that he's finally gone to sleep!
- Take a nap whenever you can while your baby is asleep during the day.

BED SHARING AND CO-SLEEPING

Sharing your bed with your baby can make nighttime feeding easier, which is probably why mothers who sleep with their baby tend to breastfeed for longer than those who don't. However, you need to be sure he's safe, so:

- Make sure he isn't overdressed and there's nothing that could cover his head. The risk of overheating comes from your baby's clothes and the bedclothes, which will tend to prevent him losing heat, not from your body, which will usually help regulate his temperature.

- If there is another child in the bed, make sure an adult sleeps between the child and the baby.
- Sleep on your side, curled round your baby, with his head just below your breast. This makes feeding easier, keeps him from going into the pillows or being lain on, and lets him roll on to his back to sleep when he lets go of your breast.
- Don't leave your baby alone in your bed.

Bed sharing is NOT a good idea if:

- There is any way your baby could get trapped or injured, either in the bed or by falling out of it.
- Either you or your partner is a smoker.
- Either you or your partner might not be able to respond normally to your baby (e.g., if you are sick, or you have drunk alcohol or taken a drug or medicine that could make you sleep unusually deeply).
- You have a saggy mattress or a waterbed, which could cause your baby to end up in a dip.
- Your baby was born early and has not yet reached his due date, or he is sick (meaning that he may not be able to alert you if he is in trouble).
- There are pets in or on the bed.

Even if you don't plan for your baby to stay in your bed after his feedings, it's best to make sure the environment is safe, just in case you fall asleep.

Note: **Sleeping with your baby in an armchair or on a couch is very dangerous.** Babies can wriggle or fall into gaps or under cushions and become wedged or covered. If you feel tired and want to lie down to breastfeed during the day, your bed is a safer place than the couch.

"I couldn't believe how much more sleep I got when I started lying down to nurse and letting Rhian stay in the bed. For the first eight weeks I'd sit upright to feed her at night and then insist on putting her back in the crib. It was counterproductive because it meant we were both awake and unsettled for longer. I had to wake up properly for each feeding and she never wanted to go back in the crib, so she was always hard to settle. I think I would have died of tiredness if I hadn't figured it out."

Amy, mother of Rhian, 14 months

Why a Bottle Isn't the Answer

Partners are often encouraged to help new mothers by doing the "night feeding." This is a great way for parents to share the care of a bottle-fed baby, but taking over a night feeding for a breastfeeding mother is *not* helpful and can lead to all sorts of extra problems, especially if the baby is given formula. Here's why:

- Replacing a breastfeeding with a bottle will affect your milk production. Cutting out nighttime nursing can mean you don't produce enough milk for your baby.
- Missing a breastfeeding can lead to engorgement and possibly even mastitis (see Chapter 13). This is a risk even if the replacement feeding is previously expressed breast milk.
- If your baby is still learning to breastfeed, giving him a bottle may mean he struggles to latch on next time, leading to an increased risk of soreness for you and frustration for you both.
- If your baby is starting to have a longer period of sleep at night, replacing a feeding at the beginning or end of it could lead to a very long gap between breastfeeds, increasing the risk of problems still further.

Some parents switch to formula in the hope of getting more sleep, only to find that although feedings happen less often, they tend to be more disruptive and tiring. Or they discover that their baby wasn't waking because he was hungry—he just needed comfort and reassurance. Without breastfeeding, they have to find another way to soothe him back to sleep. And without breastfeeding, getting back to sleep may be harder for you, too. So although it may be tempting to give a bottle at night, providing your baby is right next to you, you'll probably find it's easier to nurse him.

Breastfeeding When You're Out and About

One of the advantages of breast milk is that it's the perfect "fast food" for your baby: You always have it ready at the right temperature, so you can spend time away from home without having to plan for feedings. This makes going out and traveling much easier. However, it's common to feel uncomfortable about breastfeeding when there are other people around, especially the first time.

Nursing in public doesn't mean you have to expose your breasts—there are plenty of things you can do to make nursing discreet. Many mothers breastfeed in stores and cafés and on trains and buses all over the United States without anyone being aware of what they are doing.

In the early weeks, having a babymoon (see page 68) provides a great opportunity to get skilled at breastfeeding without anyone watching you. Practicing undoing a nursing bra with one hand and feeding with your eyes closed can help you do it by feel. It's also worth learning how to nurse in a sling and experimenting with alternative ways of holding your baby for breastfeeding (see Chapter 3) and with different types of clothes (see page 16 and page 48). **If you're nervous about how much flesh people might see, try**

feeding in front of a mirror (or your partner or a friend); most women are surprised to realize how little is revealed.

Once you and your baby have had plenty of practice at breast-feeding (and he has developed better control of his head and neck), he'll be able to latch on quickly and you won't have to look at what he's doing or fumble with your clothes. Your baby will be able to nurse tucked out of sight inside your (loose) T-shirt or sweater; under a shawl, baby blanket, or burp cloth; or in a sling. (It's worth checking before you leave the house that whatever you are wearing will be easy for breastfeeding—lifting up a dress can be awkward!)

It may help to be with someone else the first time you go out with your baby (an experienced breastfeeding friend can be reassuring) and to find a quiet spot to feed, in case he takes a while to latch on. In cafés and restaurants, you can ask for a booth or corner table if you want some privacy. You may want to check on local parenting forums for places that are popular with other nursing mothers.

As your baby gets older and becomes increasingly interested in what's going on around him, he is likely to come off the breast now and then while he's feeding—perhaps to smile at you or to watch other people. If you don't want anyone to see your breast when this happens, you'll need to move your T-shirt quickly, or grab a burp cloth to cover up. He may want to play with your clothes or stroke your other breast. If this bothers you, try giving him something else to play with (a necklace can work well) or gently holding his hand as he feeds.

Although there are occasionally stories in the press about nursing mothers being asked to leave public areas, in reality it is not that common. It's legal to breastfeed in public everywhere in the United States, and women have the right to breastfeed in any federal building or on federal property (such as museums, agencies, and national parks). However, legal protection for mothers nursing in public—in privately owned malls and restaurants, for example—varies enormously from state to state (see "Sources of Information and Support," page 291).

> "Phoebe needed to nurse the other night when we were in a restaurant with my in-laws. They said: "Can't you wait till you get home?" But they were absolutely fine about it once they realized nobody could actually see anything. And I really didn't want to carry a screaming baby all the way home just to feed her."
>
> Andrea, mother of Ryan, 4 years,
> and Phoebe, 1 year

Nursing in Front of People You Know

Some women feel very uncomfortable about nursing in front of friends or members of their extended family. If you are worried about feeling self-conscious—or making someone else feel embarrassed—there are things you can do that may make the situation easier, both for you and for those around you. Letting them know that your baby is asking to feed will give them the chance to find something else to do, at least while your baby is latching on. Or you may find that maintaining eye contact, chatting, and simply getting on with it is easiest all round. If you prefer to be discreet, try some of the tips on pages 121 and 122. Most people will take their cue from you—if you are relaxed about nursing, they are likely to relax, too, even if they haven't seen much breastfeeding before.

> "My brother came to stay when Charlotte was about five weeks old. I thought seeing me nursing her might be difficult for him because no one in our family had breastfed. At first whenever Charlotte was feeding he spent the whole time talking to me while staring at the ceiling. But she nursed so often, after a day he stopped noticing."
>
> Melissa, mother of Charlotte, 3 years

Getting Support from Others

Looking after a mother during the first few weeks so she can concentrate on her baby and on breastfeeding can make all the difference to how quickly she adapts to caring for the new member of the family. However, many people seem to expect mothers to be back to normal and doing everything they did before in a matter of days, which can make breastfeeding much more challenging than it should be.

Although the first couple of weeks are particularly crucial (which is why a babymoon is so valuable), most mothers continue to need help for several more weeks while they adjust their lifestyle to accommodate their baby. But it needs to be the right sort of help.

How Family and Friends Can Help You

It can be hard for parents and other relatives who are used to formula feeding to understand why it's important for you to stay close to your baby and feed him whenever he asks. They may want to help by taking him away to settle him, so you can rest—or suggest that someone else give him a bottle occasionally, to give you a break. These offers of help are well meant but they can seriously undermine breastfeeding.

> "My mother-in-law told me she found a pacifier a really useful way to keep her babies quiet if they woke up too early for a feeding. I don't want to use a pacifier but I didn't want to start an argument, so I just said, 'Really? Thanks—I'll remember that.' She hasn't mentioned it again."
>
> Ashley, mother of Oliver, 2 weeks

Some mothers find the answer is to have a breastfeeding "buddy" to encourage them and make it easier to turn down inappropriate offers of help, and to provide support through any breastfeeding problems. Your buddy could be your partner, your mother, a close friend, or even another nursing mother you've only just met (see below).

One of the best ways friends and relatives can support you is to boost your confidence and respect your ability to choose what's right for your baby. While there will probably be times when you *do* want someone to look after him, mostly what you'll need is for others to make you snacks and drinks, and take over time-consuming tasks (such as cooking, cleaning, and laundry) that keep you away from him.

Support from Other Mothers

There may be times when you need specific help with a breastfeeding problem, but there may also be times when you just want to meet other nursing mothers to exchange tips on everyday things, such as nighttime nursing or dealing with teething. A breastfeeding support group can provide both types of help in an informal and friendly environment.

The availability of breastfeeding support groups varies enormously and you may find you need to travel some distance to get to one, especially if you live in a rural area. Most are run by volunteers with training in breastfeeding support and counseling. Some maternity departments, birthing centers, and health centers run drop-in breastfeeding clinics that double up as support groups. Your midwife or physician should know what's available near you. Alternatively, you could contact La Leche League (see "Sources of Information and Support," page 290) to find out whether it has a group in your area.

If you can't get to a group—or don't want to—you may be able to access the support or information you need by talking to someone on a breastfeeding helpline. These are run by breastfeeding supporters or nursing mothers' counselors who can help with specific problems as well as providing a listening ear for mothers who are finding breastfeeding challenging and who simply want to vent.

What to Expect as Your Baby Gets Older

Breastfeeding changes and evolves as babies grow and mature. Mostly, these changes happen so gradually that you won't notice them until you look back, but it may be handy to know what to expect.

What to Expect with Your Breasts

The amount of milk you make when you're breastfeeding is never static—your body responds to your baby's needs as they change. Once the learning period of the first few weeks is over, your breasts settle down to make what they're being asked to make, with just a bit to spare. Then, if they get a clear message that a different quantity is needed, they start to increase or decrease production.

The way your breasts feel will change as your baby grows. For the first few weeks, they'll tend to feel full before a feeding and softer afterward. By about three months, as well as being less prone to leaking, they'll be noticeably softer most of the time. In fact, between feedings they'll probably feel like they did before you were pregnant.

This change shows that your breasts are now so in tune with your baby that they make milk extra rapidly when he is nursing and more slowly at other times. It's *not* a sign that your milk is "drying up." If your three-month-old is happy and growing, soft breasts are a sign of how well breastfeeding is going.

Adapting as Your Baby Gets Bigger

As your baby grows, you'll need to start adjusting the way you hold him for breastfeeding in order to accommodate his longer legs and body. For example, if you have been used to cradling him at your breast with your hand cupping his bottom, you may begin to find you can't reach that far—or that, if you do, his head is in the wrong position for feeding. You'll also need to figure out a different way to support him so you don't have all of his weight on your arm (and if you've been using a pillow, you'll probably find it's making things more difficult). If you don't allow for his changing size, you may find that either your baby or your breast is getting squashed, which can lead to soreness, blocked ducts, or mastitis for you, and frustration for him.

Many mothers instinctively solve the problem of holding a bigger baby by crossing their legs so that they can support their baby's bottom on their thigh, allowing their hand to move up to his rib cage. The important thing is to experiment a bit and wriggle around until you find what works for you, rather than feeling you have to stick to a particular position. As he gets bigger still, he'll become more agile and will be able to adapt his own position. (See page 174 for more on feeding older babies.)

If Your Baby Gets Distracted

As your baby gets older, he'll be increasingly interested in what's going on around him, which may mean he's easily distracted while he's feeding. He might pull away from the breast when he hears someone talking, or twist his head around (sometimes taking your nipple with him!) to look at the dog or the TV. This is fine if you've got plenty of time, but if you need him to finish nursing quickly, it could be frustrating.

If you want your baby to concentrate on breastfeeding, finding a quiet space to nurse, turning off the TV, making the room dark, and talking soothingly or singing to him will all help. If you're out, draping a burp cloth or scarf over his head and face (or feeding him tucked up inside your T-shirt) will prevent other people's movements from catching his eye.

What Happens When My Baby Is Teething?

At some point during his first year your baby's teeth will begin to appear. The teeth themselves won't affect breastfeeding (because it's his tongue, not his gums, that squeezes out the milk), but he may decide to give your breast a little bite, especially if his gums are itchy.

If your baby does decide to bite you, it will usually happen at the end of a feeding. Because his tongue covers his lower gum while he's nursing, he'll need to move it back so he doesn't bite that, too, and he can't do this while he's feeding. (He is likely to know what will hurt *him*—but he won't understand what's likely to hurt *you*.) You'll soon learn to recognize when he's starting to do this, either by feeling his attachment alter or by detecting a change in his expression. This will allow you to gently remove him from your breast before he has a chance to bite.

> "All of mine tried to bite me—but they only did it once or twice. I'm not sure whether that was because I learned to spot the gleam in their eye just before they did it, or because they were so stunned by the shriek I let out the first time that they didn't dare risk it again! Either way, it wasn't an issue for long."
>
> Bryony, mother of Patrick, 14 years, Freddie, 12 years, and Amy, 10 years

If Your Baby Goes on Strike

Occasionally a baby will refuse to breastfeed for no apparent reason. If he's very young, the most likely explanation is that he is being held awkwardly (see page 105). But if he suddenly refuses to nurse after a period of breastfeeding with no problems, it may be that he is having a nursing strike.

In a child of 18 months or older, a nursing strike may (or may not) mean that he is ready to stop breastfeeding for good. But this is very unlikely to be the case for a younger child, especially a baby under a year old, who is still reliant on milk. There are many things that can make a baby decide he doesn't want to be at the breast. For example:

- His mother's body tensed or jerked, or she gripped him suddenly while nursing. If he's teething, maybe he bit her, which made her jump.
- An older child bit or smacked him while he was breastfeeding.
- Someone close by shouted or made a sudden loud noise during a feeding.
- Breastfeeding hurts him; for example, if he has an earache or is teething.
- The milk suddenly tastes unpleasant. This could be because his mother has eaten an unfamiliar, strongly flavored food or it may be that she is starting a period, pregnant (see page 178), or developing mastitis (see page 247), all of which can change the taste of the breast milk.
- He doesn't recognize his mother. (A radical change of hairstyle, an unusually croaky voice, or an unfamiliar perfume can sometimes be enough to confuse a baby.)

If your baby has gone on strike, the first thing to do is figure out why it's happening, and if you can, stop or avoid the cause. However, sometimes there's no obvious explanation or the trigger was a random event that appears to have had a lasting effect. In this case, the best option is to concentrate on helping your baby to rediscover your chest as a lovely, soothing place to be (see below). Nursing will probably follow naturally, once he realizes that nothing horrible is going to happen.

OUCH—THAT HURTS!

Mothers are sometimes advised to breastfeed their baby while he is given an injection or has blood taken, to soothe him and take his mind off the pain. This is okay occasionally, but if your baby is having a series of injections or blood tests and discovers that every time he starts to feed he gets a sharp pain in his arm, leg, or foot, he may decide that breastfeeding hurts and it's not worth the risk. It may be better to nurse him *after* the shot rather than during it.

Helping Your Baby Get Back to Breastfeeding

The best way to help your baby overcome a suspicion of the breast is to tap into the instincts that were strongest for him when he was born. To help re-create that special time and make him feel safe:

- Make sure the room is nice and warm.
- Pull the curtains or dim the lights.
- Choose either quiet, soft music, white noise, or "womb music."

- Lie back and place your baby tummy-down on top of you, skin to skin. His head can be well away from your breasts—if he wants to feed, he'll wriggle into a nursing position by himself.
- He may cry at first; talk to him gently to help soothe him.
- Using a little warmed baby oil, massage his back, arms, and legs with long, slow, downward strokes.
- Stay in this position as long as you can, even if he falls asleep. Babies often feed instinctively when they are just drifting off or waking up. (Holding your baby skin to skin while he naps will help him feel safe against your chest.)
- Concentrate on rebuilding your relationship with your baby; feeding will follow.

Sharing a warm, relaxing bath may also help. Make sure the bathroom is warm and ask someone else to pass your baby to you once you're in the water. Lean back and lay him on your front, then pour water over him to keep him warm. A washcloth over his back will help spread the warmth evenly, so it doesn't startle him.

It's better if your baby is *not* desperately hungry when you try these ideas. If necessary, offer him a small feeding of expressed breast milk before you start, preferably in a juice glass or a sippy cup. Don't expect him to latch on and feed right away. In fact, if he's been refusing the breast for a few days, it may take more than one session before he feels confident enough to try. If he has been using a pacifier, you may want to stop this, at least temporarily, to encourage him to rediscover your breast as a source of comfort. For an older baby, meeting up with other breastfeeding mothers and babies and seeing them nursing might just remind him of what he's missing. Above all, don't rush him.

KEY POINTS

- Routines imposed by adults don't work for breastfeeding. Your baby's unique nursing pattern will emerge if you allow it to.
- Breastfeeding will get easier as you and your baby become more skilled and your breasts settle down to match his needs.
- It's easy to breastfeed discreetly if you need to when you're out and about.
- Friends and relatives can help you best by relieving you of other responsibilities, not by taking over the care of your baby.
- Other nursing mothers can be a huge source of information and support, especially while you and your baby are settling in to breastfeeding.
- The way your baby breastfeeds, and how you hold him for nursing, will evolve as breastfeeding progresses, and your breasts will feel less full most of the time.
- A period of breast refusal (or a nursing strike) doesn't necessarily mean the end of breastfeeding.

8

Lifestyle and Breastfeeding

THERE ARE ALL sorts of myths about breastfeeding, especially in relation to eating, drinking, smoking, exercise, and sex. Mostly, to breastfeed you don't need to make any changes to the things you enjoy, but there are a few that can have an impact, either on your general health or on how calm and healthy your baby is. This chapter aims to give you the facts about everyday lifestyle choices and breastfeeding.

What to Eat When You're Breastfeeding

Many people imagine that you need to eat a special diet or avoid certain foods to breastfeed. This isn't true.

Whether you eat an ideal diet is very unlikely to have any effect on your breast milk because your breasts take what your baby needs from your body stores. In countries throughout the world, women nourish their babies perfectly even though their own diet is poor—it's the mother's health that suffers first. However, giving birth and adjusting to life with a newborn are tiring. So, although you don't have to eat well to breastfeed, eating nothing but junk food will affect your energy levels and general well-being and may make looking after your baby harder.

tip

Following your baby's lead with breastfeeding helps your body rhythms match hers, so you may find you naturally want to eat and drink when she does. Make sure you have something handy to snack on whenever she nurses. If you make yourself a lunchbox first thing in the morning, you can grab it in the middle of the day. It's a good idea to keep a stock of nutritious "fast foods," such as yogurts, cheese, nuts, and fruit, in the house.

EATING FOR TWO?

You don't need to "eat for two" when you're breastfeeding because your metabolism makes better use of what you're already eating. There's no need to make a point of drinking extra water (or other fluids) to "make milk," either. Your body will put your baby's needs first and simply adjust your appetite to tell you how much you need to make up for what it has used. Many women find they naturally want to eat or drink more when they're breastfeeding (especially if they have twins), but others don't notice any difference. If you don't eat and drink *enough* you may feel fatigued, but (provided your baby feeds effectively and frequently) you will still produce plenty of milk. Eating and drinking *more* than your body is telling you it needs won't change how you feel *or* how much milk you make. All you need do is to eat and drink according to how hungry or thirsty you feel.

It's not necessary to drink milk or eat meat to make nutritious breast milk. However, mothers who eat a vegan or macrobiotic diet that contains *no* animal protein (i.e., no meat, fish, eggs, or dairy foods) should take supplements of vitamin B_{12} to be sure that they and their baby get enough of this important vitamin.

There aren't any foods that should be avoided by every breast-feeding mother. In fact, most babies actively enjoy strong flavors, such as garlic, in breast milk. The only foods you shouldn't eat are those you may have been advised to avoid because of severe allergies in the family (although so far there is no clear evidence to show that this will definitely help prevent your baby from developing allergies later).

Mothers sometimes wonder, if their baby is unusually fussy for a few hours, whether the cause might be something they ate. For example, cabbage and baked beans are often blamed for giving babies gas. But it's the roughage in these foods that causes gas—and roughage can't get into your bloodstream, or your milk. Carbonated drinks can sometimes make babies irritable, but it's the caffeine in them that's to blame (see below), not the bubbles. If you think something you've eaten may have upset your baby, avoid that food for a few days, then test it by eating it once or twice more (with a few days' gap each time) before you decide to cut it from your diet.

Caffeine passes into breast milk, and because it's a stimulant, it may make your baby irritable. It doesn't get into the milk in great quantities but it stays in a baby's system longer than it does in an adult's, so the levels can build up. While the occasional soft drink or cup of coffee may give *you* a quick buzz, having too many could end up making your baby unsettled over a longer period. Generally, fewer than five cups of coffee a day is probably okay, but every baby is different. If your baby seems miserable for no apparent reason, try cutting down your caffeine intake for a week or so to see if it helps.

Very occasionally, a baby who is constantly miserable or has a persistent rash seems to get better if her mother stops eating a particular food (e.g., dairy foods). If you suspect your baby may be reacting to a fundamental part of your diet, it's best to consult a doctor or dietitian before making big changes.

Do I Need Extra Vitamin D?

The production of vitamin D is triggered by sunlight, and exposing your skin to a reasonable amount of sun should normally allow you to make what you need. However, the lack of strong sunlight throughout the year in more northerly states, and the regular use of high-factor sunscreens in those farther south, means that many adults and children are at risk of vitamin D inadequacy. The risk is greater still for those who:

- have dark skin
- wear clothing that prevents their skin being exposed to sunlight
- rarely go outside the house
- have a body mass index (BMI) of 30 or over

For these reasons, women who are pregnant or breastfeeding are advised to take a vitamin D supplement. The American Academy of Pediatrics also recommends that all breastfed babies be given a vitamin D supplement from soon after birth. (Infant formula has the supplement already added, so additional doses are not needed until the baby is no longer reliant on formula.) Ask your health-care provider for advice.

Can I Drink Alcohol?

Small amounts are okay, but alcohol can interfere with the let-down reflex, so your baby may get slightly less milk than usual while it's in your system. But, provided you don't drink frequently, she will easily make up for this at her next few feeds. Alcohol also passes into breast milk, so it will have similar effects on your baby to those it has on you. However, her liver is immature and less able than yours to deal with it, so while the occasional single drink is unlikely to cause her any harm, anything more than this could be risky.

Although alcohol gets into breast milk, it also leaves it, with time. This is useful to know, especially if you want to have more than the occasional single drink. The level of alcohol in your milk rises at the same rate as the level in your bloodstream (peaking around thirty to sixty minutes later) and subsides as your blood level goes down, taking about three hours for a single unit of alcohol to be completely out of your system.

If you want to have a drink but prefer to minimize the effect on your baby, here's what to do:

- Offer your baby a feeding immediately *before* you have your drink.
- Have something to eat with your drink to help keep your blood alcohol level low.
- Try not to nurse your baby for at least two hours after you've finished your drink.

There's no need to express your milk and throw it away (or "pump and dump") to get rid of the alcohol; your body will deal with it naturally, in its own time.

The more you drink, the more time the alcohol will take to leave your system. **If you're planning an evening with several**

drinks, it's a good idea to express some milk during the day, so that you (or someone else) can give this expressed milk to your baby later. You will probably find you need to express some milk during the evening, too, to stay comfortable, but this is for *your* benefit, not your baby's. It won't affect the amount of alcohol she gets at her next feed—only time will do that.

> "Lots of my friends who've had babies don't breastfeed because they think they won't be able to drink or go out. But I didn't want to go out all the time anyway after I had Lucia. And when I did I'd express some milk and my sister would feed her. It wasn't a big deal. Now my friends have seen the comfort she gets from the breast and how easy it is, they say they'd think about it next time."
>
> Irene, mother of Lucia, 11 months

Taking Over-the-Counter Medicines

Most medicines are safe to take while breastfeeding, and an alternative is usually available for the few that aren't. The majority either don't get into breast milk or do so only in extremely small amounts. However, this isn't always clear. The leaflet that accompanies a medicine often states that it should not be taken while breastfeeding even though it can be quite safe to do so. This is because testing a drug for safety during lactation costs time and money, so not all manufacturers do it routinely.

Over-the-counter medicines such as acetaminophen, ibuprofen, antacids, and hemorrhoid treatments can all be taken at normal dosages without presenting a risk to your baby. Most asthma medications and flu vaccines are safe. However, there are some medicines to avoid:

- Decongestants (such as pseudoephedrine) can drastically reduce milk production.

- Codeine can make babies sleepy.
- Aspirin is not safe for babies and young children.
- Some hay fever remedies can make babies drowsy (eye drops and nasal sprays don't get absorbed into the blood-stream, so they are safe to use).

Some herbal remedies can also present a risk to either the baby or the milk supply, and since they are not regulated and controlled, the strength of even "safe" products is very variable. If in doubt, ask your health-care provider for advice.

There has been little research into the possible effects of dental work on breast milk, but it's thought the amount of mercury in a single filling would be too small to do any harm. The anesthetic used in routine dental work is safe, although adrenaline is some-times added to minimize bleeding and this can occasionally make a very sensitive baby irritable. Tell your dentist you are breastfeeding before planning any treatment.

You or your health-care provider can check online for informa-tion about drugs in breast milk—see "Sources of Information and Support," page 291.

Can I Go On a Diet?

Almost all mothers put on weight while they are pregnant. Some of this extra weight goes into making breast milk, so in theory your pregnancy weight should disappear gradually and consistently over the first few months. However, not all women find that this works in practice and many want to speed up the process. It used to be said that breastfeeding mothers shouldn't try to lose weight, but current evidence suggests that avoiding excess calories causes no problems for either mother or baby. Sudden crash dieting or eating fewer than 1,800 calories per day is not a good idea, though.

Is It Okay to Exercise?

Moderate exercise is a good thing for a breastfeeding mother. It helps you stay fit, gets your shape back after pregnancy, and relieves stress. In the past, it was thought that extreme exercise might make babies refuse to breastfeed because of high levels of lactic acid in the breast milk (which could make it taste odd), but research suggests this isn't a problem. In general, if exercising feels good, it's probably fine for both of you. But if it makes you very tired or dehydrated, it might be a good idea to scale it down.

What If I Smoke?

If you can't manage to give up smoking, it's *much* better for your baby to be breastfed than to have formula. Breastfeeding helps prevent illnesses such as bronchitis, pneumonia, and ear infections, which are otherwise more common in babies whose mothers smoke. **The biggest risk is from the smoke itself, not from the ingredients of smoke that make it into your milk,** so the most important thing is to avoid smoking near your baby or in the rooms in which she spends a lot of time. (To avoid smoke from clothes, some mothers keep a jacket to wear when smoking that they can take off when holding their baby.)

Breastfeeding has been shown to lower the risk of sudden infant death syndrome (crib death), but sharing a bed with a smoker is known to *increase* the risk—even if no one smokes in the bedroom. So while keeping your baby near you at night is still recommended if you or your partner smokes, having her in your bed isn't. (See page 118 for more on safe bed sharing.) Although the main risk to your baby's health is from breathing smoke, nicotine is not particularly good for her, either—and the concentration of nicotine in your milk is three times higher than it is in your blood. The best way to reduce the amount of nicotine your baby gets is to smoke immediately *after* a breastfeeding—or, if you're desperate for a cigarette, to offer her a quick feeding before you light up.

Nicotine patches are safe to use while breastfeeding. However, patches deliver a steady level of nicotine throughout the day, so the level in your milk will be constant. Use the lowest-strength patches you can to replace the amount of nicotine your body is used to. If you opt for lozenges or gum, fit them around your baby's feedings, as described above, to minimize the amount of nicotine she gets.

MARIJUANA GETS INTO BREAST MILK

The active ingredient in marijuana (cannabis) accumulates in breast milk, with the level rising to as much as eight times that in the mother's bloodstream. It is also stored in body fat, meaning it can stay in a mother's system (and in her milk) for several weeks after she last smoked (or ate) it. At the very least, it can make a baby sleepy and reluctant to feed but the long-term effects may be more serious. It is generally recommended that breastfeeding mothers avoid marijuana (and other, more dangerous street drugs). And of course, being under the influence of drugs can make you unable to care for your baby safely.

Your Sex Life

Caring for a baby can be exhausting. While some mothers say breastfeeding makes them feel extra sexy, it's not unusual for a couple's sex life to take a dive when they first become parents. But it's not just tiredness. Breastfeeding, hugging, and carrying involve a lot of physical contact, so at the end of a full-on day of mothering, it can be hard to share your body yet again. Simply having an hour or so to relax while someone else looks after the baby may help.

When you do find time for intimacy, you may need to adapt what you do to accommodate the fact that you are breastfeeding. While positions that were uncomfortable during pregnancy will now be possible again, it's likely your breasts may feel more tender than before you were pregnant, especially when they're full. In general, it will probably be more enjoyable and comfortable if you have sex just after nursing. Be ready for the "love" hormone to trigger your let-down reflex as things heat up and perhaps warn your partner that you may leak milk.

Using Breastfeeding as a Contraceptive

Breastfeeding naturally prevents a quick return to fertility to allow the mother's body to concentrate on nourishing the baby she is nursing rather than on growing a new one. As long as the baby breastfeeds frequently and has no other food or drink, the level of prolactin in the mother's bloodstream will stay high enough to override her normal menstrual cycle, preventing her from ovulating. This means that breastfeeding *can* be a reliable contraceptive, depending on the circumstances (see box on the following page).

If you are breastfeeding frequently and exclusively, you're unlikely to menstruate for at least six months after your baby is born—and possibly quite a bit longer. Some women are alerted to their first postbirth period by their baby temporarily rejecting the breast, because hormonal changes make their breast milk taste slightly different. However, this is not a reliable way of telling whether you are fertile again, since it's possible you'll ovulate for the first time *before* you have your first period. If you don't want to rely on breastfeeding to prevent you becoming pregnant again, or if your baby is older than six months, it's advisable to use another method, too.

Most contraceptive methods that involve hormones, such as the combined pill or injections, can reduce breast milk production, although some mothers find they can start taking the mini pill after the first six weeks without a problem. However, synthetic hormones can also be passed to the baby through breast milk, and many mothers prefer to avoid the pill for this reason. For most breastfeeding couples, a barrier method of contraception, such as a diaphragm or condoms, is a good solution. Nonhormonal types of intrauterine devices (IUDs) may be suitable, too. If you go to a doctor for contraceptive advice, be sure to let him or her know you're breastfeeding.

THE LACTATIONAL AMENORRHEA METHOD OF CONTRACEPTION (LAM)

Breastfeeding can be as reliable as other commonly used methods of contraception, provided that:

- The baby is under six months old.
- The mother hasn't had a period since her baby was born.
- The baby is having only breast milk, with no other foods or drinks (including water).
- The baby is nursing frequently, during the day and at night, with no more than one gap of longer than four hours (but not longer than six) in every twenty-four.

KEY POINTS

🔑 A mother's body looks after her baby first, so you don't need to have a perfect diet to breastfeed. But if your diet is poor, you may find caring for your baby more tiring.

- There's no need to avoid particular foods while you're breastfeeding unless you have been advised to because of allergies.
- Occasionally something in a mother's diet may make her baby unsettled. Caffeine is a common culprit.
- The occasional glass of alcohol is okay; if you want to drink more, you may need to plan ahead.
- Most over-the-counter medicines are safe to take while breastfeeding; if in doubt, check with your health-care provider, a pharmacist, or online.
- Dieting is safe while you're breastfeeding as long as it isn't too extreme or sudden.
- It's safe to exercise when you're breastfeeding as long as you don't overdo it.
- If you smoke, your baby is likely to be healthier if you breastfeed her than if you don't. Try to minimize the amount of smoke she breathes—and don't share a bed with her.
- Your breasts may be more tender during sex than they were before pregnancy, and you may leak milk.
- Breastfeeding can be a reliable contraceptive for the first six months, depending on your circumstances.

9

When You Can't Be
with Your Baby

IF THERE ARE times when you need to leave your baby with someone else, whether it's the occasional evening out or going back to work
or study full-time, breastfeeding can continue to be baby led. There's
no need to introduce bottles or get your baby into a routine for the
times when you are apart. Understanding how your milk production works is key: You can be led by your baby when you are with
him and, for the most part, by how your breasts feel when you aren't.

Frequent feeding when you're together can help make up for
the time you have to spend apart, both physically (in terms of milk
production) and emotionally, in terms of your relationship.

This chapter is about how to manage different kinds of separations so you can continue to meet your baby's needs. (The issues
will be slightly different if you and your baby are separated because
one of you is sick—see Chapter 14—or if your baby is born early
and is in a neonatal unit—see Chapter 11.)

How Can I Provide Milk for My Baby While
We Are Apart?

If you are apart from your baby for more than a couple of hours
while he's fully breastfed (i.e., younger than around six months),

you'll need to leave him some milk. The younger he is, the more you'll need to leave. The best milk for your baby is your breast milk. Milk that has been expressed within the previous twenty-four hours is ideal, because it contains active, up-to-date antibodies, but milk that has been refrigerated for three to eight days (see table on page 156) is a good alternative. Breast milk will also keep for up to six months in a freezer (see page 155), so you can build up a reserve stock in advance, if necessary. This will give you something to fall back on occasionally if you don't have enough freshly expressed.

Although each mother's milk is specifically made for her own baby, the differences between one woman's milk and the next are very small, so in terms of your baby's health, the next best thing to your breast milk is another mother's milk. Years ago, co-feeding (or "wet nursing") was widely practiced, and even today some mothers find it convenient to share breastfeeding with, for example, a sister or close friend when they can't be with their baby. If you're considering this option, check beforehand that you and your friend agree about issues such as alcohol and medicines, which your baby could be exposed to in the milk he receives, and that you both have up-to date health screening for serious infections. You'll need to make sure both your partners are happy with the arrangement, too. (There is also a growing trend to use expressed milk donated or sold through informal online milk-sharing communities, although this is currently discouraged by US health authorities because of potentially inadequate health checks and milk storage issues.)

The third option is for your baby to have formula when you can't be with him. This avoids your having to express milk in advance, but it disturbs some of the protective effects for his health of having only breast milk (and it can be expensive). However, many mothers find that, for regular separations, this is a workable choice that allows them to keep breastfeeding going. See page 158 for information on combining formula with breastfeeding.

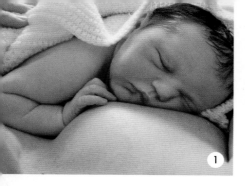
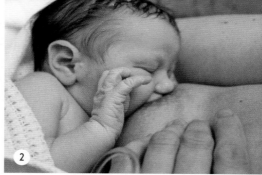

▲ As soon as she's born, Scarlett is laid skin to skin on her mother's chest. She rests a while, then finds the breast and has her first feed.

Mike helps Billie to hold their newborn twins, Ottilie and Anna, in skin contact, so they can feed as soon as they're ready (see page 54). ▼

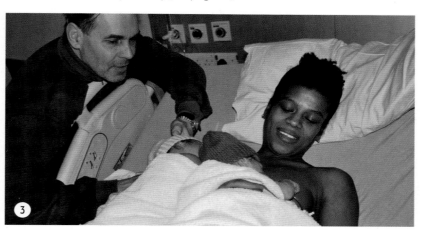

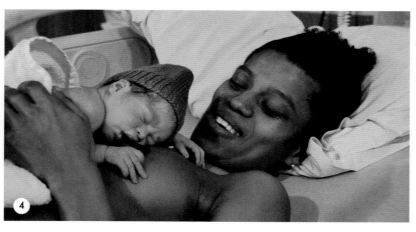

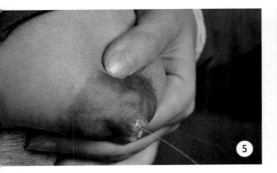

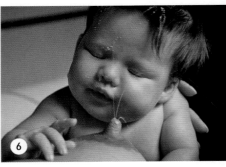

▲ Hand expressing breast milk is a useful skill and is easy once you get the knack (see page 86).

▲ Artemis is able to pull herself away from a strong let-down reflex (see page 22). She'll wait a few seconds for the flow to subside before she goes back on to the breast.

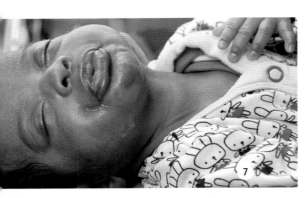

◀ Munira has finished feeding and now looks "milk drunk."

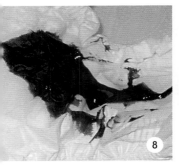

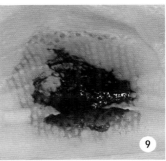

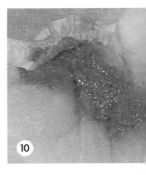

▲ These photos show a newborn baby's poop on the first, third, and fifth days after birth. The gradual change from the greenish-black, sticky meconium to yellow, runny poop shows that she is getting plenty of milk (see page 100).

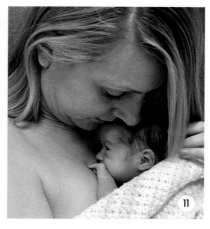

◀ Michaela holds Jacob, one of her premature twins, in kangaroo care (see page 199). Being held this way has many benefits and allows him to breastfeed as soon as he's ready.

Trudy holds newborn Noah in skin-to-skin contact on the operating table after his caesarean birth, with Derek looking on. Skin contact is the best way for breastfeeding to begin and is especially important after this type of birth (see page 62).▼

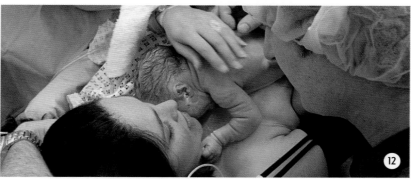

◀ If you have a blocked duct or mastitis, your baby can help to clear it by feeding in a position that targets the sore area (see page 246). Leaning over your baby to feed is especially helpful.

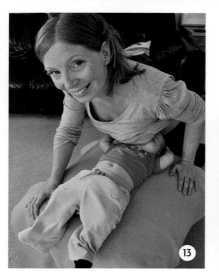

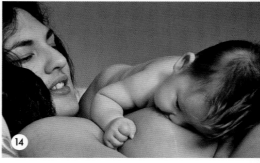

Beatrice, six weeks, approaches the breast, nose to nipple, and scoops up a big mouthful, with the nipple pointing towards the roof of her mouth. Once attached, her chin is pressing into the breast, her nose is free, her cheeks are full, and more of her mother's areola is visible above her top lip than below her bottom lip (see pages 34 and 48). When she's finished feeding she lets go of the breast and sleeps.

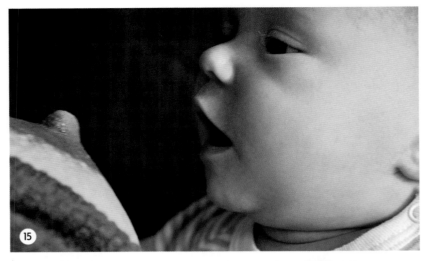

15

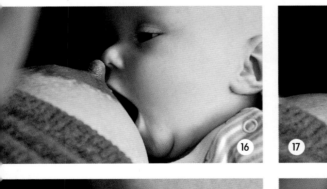

16

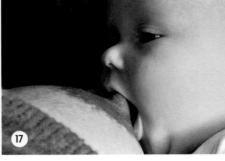

17

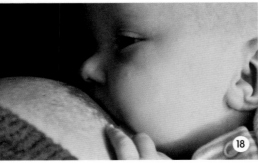

18

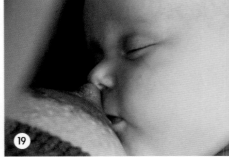

19

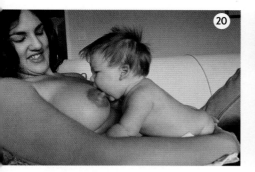

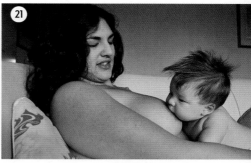

Artemis, eight weeks, shows how easily she can use her instincts when she's lying on her mother (see page 41). Her head and arms are strong enough for her to get into a position where she can easily attach, and she uses her hands to steady herself and the breast. She doesn't need any help!

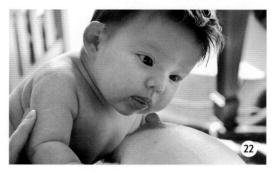

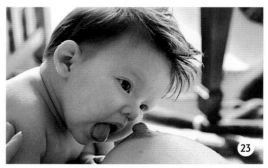

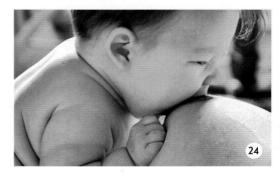

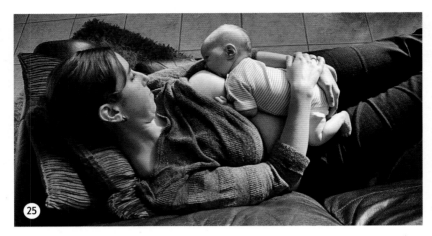

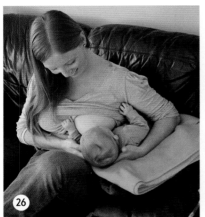

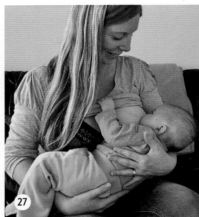

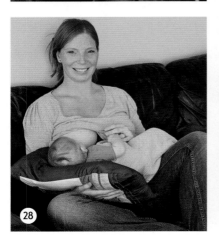

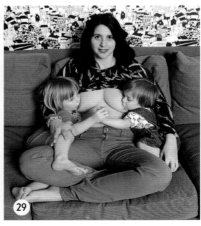

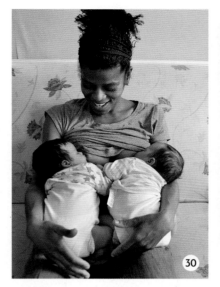

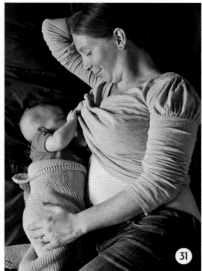

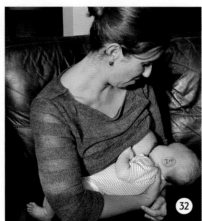

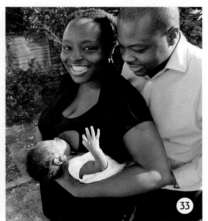

Whether you're feeding one baby or two, as long as they are in a position that makes it easy for them to feed, you can sit, stand, lie back, or lie down to breastfeed—whatever suits you and your baby (or babies).

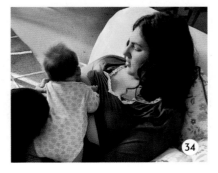

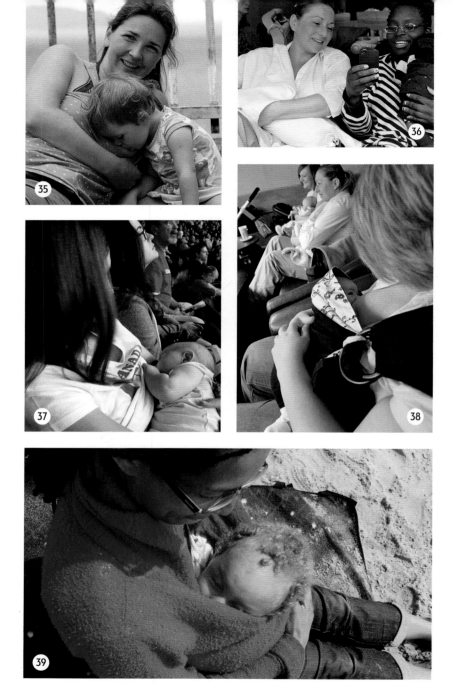

Breastfeeding is an easy way to feed your baby when you're out and about. If you want, you can cover up with your clothes, a sling, or a burp cloth.

However your baby is fed when you are not with him, you will need to express at least some breast milk while you are apart, to prevent overfullness and maintain your milk production. For brief separations you can be led by how your breasts feel. Just express enough to keep yourself comfortable—and feed your baby again as soon as you can. If the separation is longer or repeated regularly (e.g., if you are going back to work or school), expressing at roughly the times when he would usually be feeding will keep your breasts producing milk at a steady rate. **If you have to leave your baby in the first two weeks, you'll need to express frequently while you're apart so that the setting-up of your capacity for long-term milk production isn't affected.**

tip

If your baby is older than about eight months and has started eating some solid foods, he may be able to go for several hours without nursing—as long as he's able to breastfeed frequently enough to make up for it (including during the night) when you are together again.

Putting In an Advance Order for Expressed Milk

Breastfeeding works on the principle of production according to demand. So, by the time he's a few weeks old, you'll be producing as much milk as your baby needs—but not a lot more. This means that if you try to express, you may not get much at all, especially immediately after a breastfeeding. Expressing and freezing small amounts now and then is a useful way to build up a small store in case you need it unexpectedly, but if you want your breasts to make more milk on a regular basis, you'll have to give them some notice. It's all about putting in the order.

What If I Have to Leave My Baby for an Afternoon?

If you're going to be away from your baby for only a few hours, and you have a day or two's notice, you should be able to get away with expressing three or four times during that period, and storing the milk in the refrigerator (see page 155). If you haven't previously been expressing regularly, you may not be able to express enough for a really satisfying feeding, but—unless your baby is very young—this won't matter. Provided he has something to take the edge off his hunger, he'll make up for it when you're back together.

tip

If you leak milk from one breast while feeding from the other, you can collect this "drip milk" in a milk collector (see page 80) and freeze it. However, milk that leaks freely at the beginning of a breastfeeding tends to be low in fat, so a feeding consisting entirely of drip milk may not satisfy your baby's hunger for long. It's fine for the occasional short-term separation but is unlikely to be sufficient on its own for long-term use.

How Can I Prepare to Go Back to Work?

If you're going back to work or school, it's a good idea to have a reasonable store of expressed milk in your freezer as a "buffer" while you are coming to grips with the changes. This will also give you peace of mind if you go through a temporary downward "blip" in milk production, which can happen if you are exceptionally busy. It's best to start building up your store *at least* a few days before you're going to need to start using expressed milk, and preferably a few weeks.

To express and save milk in advance, you need to put in an order for more than your baby's current needs. The best way to do this is to mimic the way he asks to nurse more often during an "appetite spurt," when he needs to increase your supply. This means expressing milk regularly between feedings (especially in any longer gaps), and expressing from the second breast whenever your baby feeds only (or mainly) from one. (Expressing just after your baby has nursed can also work, although you'll probably get less out at first that way.) **Your baby is likely to be far more efficient at getting milk out of your breasts than either your hands or a breast pump will be, so don't worry if the amounts you express are small, especially at first.** Breastfed babies rarely take as much milk during a feeding (or even during a whole day) as do babies on formula, so your baby won't need or expect huge quantities. Fitting in two or three expressing sessions over twenty-four hours means your breasts will quickly get the message and start to make more. You'll probably notice a difference within a day or two: they'll feel slightly fuller and you'll be getting more milk each time. The secret, though, is to focus on putting in the order, rather than on the quantities you're getting out.

Once you go back to work or school, you should aim to express roughly as many times as your baby would have nursed (or more often). In practice, however, most mothers who work full-time don't manage to express more than about three times a day, and many get by with fewer. (See page 162 for information on expressing at work.) The key is to listen to your body and express as soon as your breasts start to feel full—and to encourage your baby to breastfeed as much as possible when you are not at work, to make up for any missed sessions.

"By about ten months, the amounts I pumped were getting smaller and smaller, probably because Poppy was drinking less during the day. I stopped expressing but carried on breastfeeding in the morning, evening and night. She'd usually have a long feeding before I went to work and she'd be on the breast lots when I was home. She just had solids during the day."

Alison, mother of Jack, 4 years,
and Poppy, 2 years

What Happens If I Need to Leave My Baby for More Than a Day?

Occasionally, mothers need to provide milk for their baby for a day or two, with only a few days' notice, perhaps because of work or social commitments or because they need to stop breastfeeding temporarily for a medical reason. If you want your baby to continue to have only your milk but you don't have a stock to fall back on, you'll need to express intensively in any available time to stockpile as much as you can.

To increase your milk production rapidly, set yourself a target of expressing as often as you possibly can, both after and between feedings, draining your breasts as fully as possible each time (see "How to Give Your Breasts a Two-Week 'Wake-up Call,'" page 195, for tips on maximizing the amount you express). Provided you don't express immediately before your baby is likely to want a big meal, you will still have enough milk for him. (If he wants to feed more often because there isn't quite as much there as usual, that will help stimulate your breasts even more.)

If the separation happens immediately after this period of intense expressing, you'll probably need to express frequently to stay comfortable (and prevent engorgement) while you and your baby are apart because of the increased production you've generated. However, if you're not aiming to save the milk (perhaps because it contains a drug that your baby mustn't have), there's no need to wash and sterilize any equipment you use during this time.

Once you and your baby are back together, it will take a little while for your needs and his to get back in sync, so don't be surprised if his usual feeding pattern takes a day or two to return.

"I went on a two-day business trip when Lola was 15 months. I took the pump with me and expressed in the hotel room to keep comfortable. I was surprised how full I got, even so—she was obviously still drinking a lot of milk, even though she wasn't having it during the day. By the time I got home the next evening my boobs felt like they were exploding. I had to wake her up to feed. She was so happy—she said 'Mommy!', then 'Booby!'"

Sam, mother of Lola, 2 years

How to Express Your Milk

You can express your milk by hand or with a pump—or you can use a combination of both methods. Hand expression (see page 87) has several advantages over pumping and, with a bit of practice, it can be just as quick. If you practice expressing by hand first, you'll be able to decide whether you need a pump. You'll need to wash your hands before expressing milk to be given to your baby.

When you feed your baby, your let-down reflex operates without you having to think about it, but when you express your milk you may find it needs a little help, especially if you're using a pump. One solution is to express from one breast while feeding your baby from the other. This works particularly well if you're very full and he is likely to want only one breast, but it can be a bit clumsy to manage at first, especially if he tends to wriggle. If you want to express when he's not breastfeeding, cuddling him skin to skin can be a good way to trigger the let-down reflex.

If you need to express and haven't got your baby near you, you can stimulate your let-down reflex in other ways. Each woman's oxytocin triggers are different, so feel free to experiment to find what works for you. Remember that oxytocin is the "love" hormone; it can easily be turned off if you don't feel relaxed, comfortable, and safe, so take some time to focus and get in the mood, if you need to. The following box contains some ideas that may help (although the ones you can use in a work environment might be limited!).

IDEAS FOR ENCOURAGING YOUR LET-DOWN REFLEX

- a photo or video of your baby
- an item of your baby's clothing (worn, so it smells of him)
- a recording of your baby squeaking or murmuring
- a warm bath, or warm washcloths laid over your breasts
- a warm drink
- relaxing music
- low lighting
- relaxation techniques—perhaps some you practiced for use in labor
- gentle breast massage or stimulation—whatever feels nice but nothing too deep. The purpose isn't to push milk down the ducts but to get your oxytocin going
- If you like, your partner can hug you, talk soothingly to you, give you a back massage, or touch and stroke your breasts.

There's no need to watch the clock when you're expressing; your milk flow is a much more useful guide as to how long you should keep going. If you're trying to get as much milk as possible, keep expressing as long as you're getting milk, then switch to the other breast. When the flow subsides on that one, switch back to the first. This will trigger a new let-down and release another rush of milk.

Expressing from both breasts at once can be very effective at triggering the let-down reflex and stimulating milk production, as well as cutting down the time you need to spend. Some electric pumps are equipped for double pumping; if you're expressing by hand, you'll find it easier, and less messy, to catch the milk if you use a really wide bowl or pitcher.

There's no advantage in continuing to express if nothing much is coming out. Switching to the other breast, doing some gentle breast massage or nipple stimulation, or simply taking a break (even for a couple of minutes) will do more to stimulate both milk flow and milk production than will keeping going when nothing is happening.

How Do I Choose a Breast Pump?

There are lots of different breast pumps on the market. If possible, talk to friends who have used a pump—perhaps even try theirs—and look on the Internet before deciding which type will suit you best. The more time you will be spending apart from your baby and the more determined you are to ensure he has only your milk, the more you will benefit from a sophisticated pump—but size and portability will be important, too.

Hand-operated pumps have either a bulb or a handle, which you squeeze to create a vacuum. The degree of suction is controlled by how hard and how long you squeeze. Electric pumps run on battery or electricity, or both, with a dial for setting your preferred strength. **Although some are quieter than others, all electric pumps make a noise when they're working—which is worth bearing in mind if you want to be able to use your pump discreetly at work!** You may want to get an adaptor so you can use the pump in your car.

All pumps come apart for cleaning and sterilizing, though some are trickier than others to reassemble.

If you need to pump intensively short term—for example, if your baby is premature or sick and has to be in the hospital (see pages 193 and 259)—you may be able to rent a pump from the hospital. If not, you can search online for your nearest pump rental station. However, if you are going back to work, it's probably cheaper and more convenient to buy your own.

The size of the flange (or funnel) can make a difference to how much milk you get. If the pump you choose comes with more than one flange, it's worth experimenting to see whether one works better than the other. It's also important to start expressing gently and build up the suction gradually until you find the intensity that's best for you. Strong suction isn't necessarily good or effective, so there's no need to feel you have to get to the maximum setting.

Follow the manufacturer's instructions for how to set up, dismantle, clean, and sterilize the various parts of your pump.

tip

A few minutes of hand expression before you start pumping can help get your hormones—and your milk—flowing. Another bit of hand expressing afterward can help you get more of the thick, creamy milk that comes as the breast is being drained.

How to Store Breast Milk

The recommendations in this section refer to milk that is being stored for a healthy baby to drink in a home environment or day nursery. See Chapter 11 for what to do if your baby is in a neonatal unit.

Breast milk can be stored in a feeding bottle, a specially designed sterile bag, or a food-safe plastic container that has been thoroughly cleaned and then scalded with boiling water. Unlike formula, it doesn't spoil easily because it contains living cells that stop bacteria multiplying, so it can be stored safely for quite long periods.

At normal room temperature, breast milk will be safe for six hours—and it can be kept for about eight hours in a cool bag with ice packs. (Make sure the ice packs don't touch the milk container so the milk doesn't freeze.) **There's no need to refrigerate milk you express to be given to your baby within a few hours.**

Breast milk will keep for about a week in a refrigerator that is at a constant temperature of less than 39°F. However, most domestic refrigerators aren't kept that low. Three days is fine as long as the temperature doesn't rise above 50°F. Keep the milk at the back of the refrigerator rather than in the door, to be sure.

Breast milk can be stored in a freezer (at a temperature of 0°F or lower) for up to six months. Saving it in small amounts will make it easier and less wasteful to defrost. Each new batch should be frozen separately rather than added to a container that already has frozen milk in it. Label each one with the date of expressing.

Frozen breast milk is best defrosted slowly, in a refrigerator, and used within twelve hours. If you need it more quickly than this, defrost it by standing the container in hand-hot water and shaking it gently every few minutes. Fully defrosted breast milk should be used immediately. Freezing and defrosting can cause milk to separate, but that doesn't mean it's not safe to use; a quick, gentle shake is all that's needed to mix the cream back in. However, if the milk smells sour, throw it away—and don't refreeze milk that's been defrosted.

There's no need to heat breast milk before offering it to your baby—and *over*heating it may destroy some of the protective antibodies. However, many babies don't like milk right from the fridge, in which case taking it out half an hour before you need it, or warming it slightly by standing the bottle or container in a bowl of hand-hot water for a minute or two, is all that's needed. **Never heat breast milk in a microwave oven or a saucepan—you risk overheating it and destroying some of its valuable ingredients, as well as possibly scalding your baby's mouth.**

QUICK GUIDE TO STORING BREAST MILK

WHERE/WHAT TEMPERATURE	MILK WILL KEEP FOR UP TO:
Room temperature	6 hours
Cool bag with ice packs	8 hours
Refrigerator (maximum temp. 50°F)	3 days
Refrigerator (maximum temp. 39°F)	8 days
Freezer (maximum temp. 0°F)	6 months

Should I Introduce a Bottle?

Nursing mothers are sometimes advised to get their baby used to a bottle as early as possible so that he will accept one later. However, introducing a bottle when your baby is still learning to breastfeed can cause problems. Feeding from a bottle is different from breastfeeding (see page 32), and he may find it difficult to switch between one and the other if he is asked to learn both at the same time. (Contrary to what some advertisements say, there is no bottle on sale that is really "like a breast" because your breast molds itself to the shape of your baby's mouth when he feeds and changes shape as he sucks and swallows.) For short separations, it may be better to feed a very young baby with a small cup (see box).

If you do decide to use a bottle while your baby is still very

HOW TO FEED A YOUNG BABY USING A CUP

Cup feeding is a useful way to give small amounts of milk to a baby who is still learning to breastfeed so that he can avoid using a bottle. The cup needs to be small to reduce the risk of accidental choking. A shot glass, medicine cup, egg cup, or the cover from a feeding bottle are all about the right size. Check that the rim is smooth and rounded and not too thick. Wash the cup in hot, soapy water and rinse it well.

To cup feed a baby:

- Fill the cup about three quarters full to start with, so it won't spill easily but won't need to be tipped too much, either.
- Wrap the baby so his arms can't knock the cup and cause the milk to spill.
- Sit him upright on your lap, with the heel of your hand on his upper back.
- Support his neck with the fingers and thumb of the same hand, so that he can lift his chin slightly.
- Rest the cup gently on the baby's lower lip and tilt it so that the milk touches his upper lip.
- Wait for him to start lapping or sipping. *Don't be tempted to pour milk into his mouth, because that could make him choke.*
- Leave the cup in place, adjusting the tilt to keep the milk touching the baby's top lip.
- Let him take the milk at his own pace. It's important that the baby is in control of the feeding. (Be prepared for his trying to suck, which may be messy.)
- Be ready to add more milk to the cup when it gets down to about a quarter full.

young, try to ensure that whoever is feeding him coaxes him to use the same sort of technique he needs to use for breastfeeding, rather than poking the bottle into his mouth. Touching the bottle against his nose will encourage him to open his mouth wide and stick his tongue out, so that he "scoops" it up. This will help him remember what to do when he's breastfeeding.

Babies who are efficient at breastfeeding can generally figure out how to use a bottle and will switch back to the breast without difficulty. And babies older than six months (some as young as four months) are usually able to manage a small glass or a sippy cup by themselves, in which case there's no need to introduce a bottle at all.

Cups, bottles, and bottle nipples need to be thoroughly cleaned in hot, soapy water, and rinsed in clear water after each feeding (the top rack of the dishwasher is fine for this). It's a good idea to sterilize bottles and nipples once a day by boiling for ten minutes or using a steam sterilizer, or in a specially designed bag in the microwave. Cups are easier than bottles to clean and dry thoroughly, so the risk of germs multiplying is less and sterilizing isn't necessary. If your baby is premature or at particular risk of infection, be advised by your health-care provider about whether, and how often, you need to sterilize feeding equipment.

What If I Decide to Use Formula?

If you decide that your baby will have formula when you can't be with him, there are a few things it may be useful to know about which formula to choose and how to prepare it.

A proprietary infant formula (not Step 2 or toddler formula) is the best substitute for breast milk. Most brands come in ready-to-feed, concentrated, or powdered form. Ready-to-feed and concentrated formulas are convenient, and sterility is guaranteed, but they tend to be expensive. Powdered formula is generally cheaper, but it is not necessarily sterile, even when the box or can has only just been opened. **Adding water to the powder allows any bacteria in the milk to start reproducing, so powdered formula should be made up freshly for each feeding, not prepared in advance.** Make sure your baby's caretaker knows how to prepare the formula (see box).

If your baby has followed a typical breastfeeding pattern, you may find that he prefers to stick to small, frequent feedings and that he needs less formula at each feeding than the instructions on the container suggest. It's important to explain this to whoever is looking after him. If he has not previously been given any bottles, persuading him to accept one may take gentleness and perseverance (see page 160). If he is older than four or five months, he may prefer an open cup or sippy cup to a bottle.

HOW TO PREPARE A BOTTLE OF FORMULA

If your baby is going to be fed using an open cup or sippy cup with no quantity markings on the side, the formula will need to be made up in a clean feeding bottle (or other container) and then transferred to the cup.

To prepare formula:

- Use recently boiled tap water (not bottled water, which can be high in salt).
- Measure the right amount of water into the bottle.
- Using the scoop provided, add the correct amount of powder, leveling off the scoop with a flat edge (such as the back of a knife blade).
- Shake well to mix the formula.
- Cool to a safe temperature, preferably under running cold water.
- Throw away any unused formula.

What If My Baby Refuses to Be Fed?

Some babies won't accept feedings from bottles or cups, and this can make separations stressful for everyone concerned. Partners and grandparents can feel hurt and anxious if they can't persuade the baby to eat, while knowing your baby won't take a feeding from anyone else may make leaving him extra difficult for you. Offering before the baby is truly hungry can sometimes help, but trying to force a baby to feed when he is clearly saying no is likely to lead to more problems, not fewer.

> "I went back to work when Ava was six months and I was really worried because she refused to have a bottle or a cup. I thought she'd starve. Right up until the day I started work I didn't know what would happen. But on the first day, our nanny gave her a bottle and just let her play with it. She eventually figured it out for herself. The nanny wasn't worried—she knew Ava would discover what to do as she'd done it with lots of other babies. So she was fine from the first day."
>
> Tania, mother of Ava, 18 months

Babies don't starve themselves—they will eat if they need to. Many breastfeeding babies whose mothers are at work or school decide to manage without milk while Mommy isn't there—and make up for it by feeding frequently when she is. And many breastfeeding mothers are more than happy to spend time catching up on their relationship with their baby when they are back together.

If your baby decides to go on a feeding strike during the day and make up for lost time at night, you will probably want to make sure nursing at night is as easy as possible for both of you—see page 117 for some tips. You may need to be prepared to allow extra time in the mornings for your baby to have a good feeding before you leave him and to spend most of the evening with him at your breast.

Whether or not your baby is happy to be fed by someone else, being fed with a bottle or cup won't feel the same to him as breast-feeding, so it's important that his caretaker holds him close during the feeding and gives him plenty of affection.

How Do I Manage Going Back to Work?

Many women make their decision about the best time to go back to work or school when they are pregnant. However, with your first baby it can be hard to predict how the separation will affect your nursing relationship. In general, the longer you can delay your return, the easier it will be—there's no doubt that going back when your baby is as young as six weeks, for example, will be very challenging for both of you. However, by the time he is three months, he will have established his feeding pattern and nursing him won't take as long, which will give you more time for expressing. From six months onward, he may well be having some solid foods as well, so he won't be totally reliant on breast milk. This will make it easier for others to share his care.

> "I'm really glad Martha was still nursing when I went back to work. The separation would have been much harder if I'd stopped breastfeeding at the same time. Because I was still nursing her we could bond again in the evening and at night-time—that was really important for both of us."
>
> Beth, mother of Martha, 15 months

If commuting with your baby is a practical option, choosing a daycare center near your work or school rather than near your home will shorten the time you have to spend away from him. This can mean you don't have to miss as many feedings, and you may even be able to breastfeed during your lunch break.

If you want to nurse your baby at lunch and/or when you pick him up, make sure his caretaker knows when you will arrive, and ask her not to give him a full feeding just before you get there. If your baby is being cared for by a relative or nanny (rather than at daycare), ask if she can bring him to your workplace at lunch so you can feed him there.

It's easy when bottle feeding (or spoon feeding) to persuade a baby to take more than he needs, which can disrupt his usual breastfeeding pattern. If possible, explain to your baby's caretaker that he is used to deciding how much he needs and that small feed-ings (or just a little solid food) are fine with you. It may be worth explaining that formula-fed babies almost always require more milk than breastfed babies do because formula contains ingredients that can't be fully digested.

It's a good idea to have a few days' trial run with your child-care arrangements before you return to work or school so you can iron out any issues in advance. This will help you feel more relaxed and confident on your first day back.

Tips for Expressing at Work

Expressing milk for your baby while you are at work takes a bit of planning. Many mothers find they have more milk at the beginning of their working week than toward the end, so they focus on expressing milk most intensively in the first few days. Having something with you that reminds you of your baby will help you get your let-down reflex to work (see "Ideas for Encouraging Your Let-Down Reflex," page 152). And you may find it useful to keep a supply of wet wipes, breast pads, and a spare top and bra at work, in case of leaks.

Employers are bound by legislation to do what they can

to enable mothers to keep breastfeeding for the first year of a baby's life.

Your employer must allow you breaks for expressing, and provide you with privacy and a clean and safe place (*not* a bathroom) to express and store your milk. You may be able to negotiate the use of a refrigerator, although a cool bag with ice packs will do instead (see page 155). See "Sources of Information and Support," page 290, for details of organizations that can provide further information on your rights as a breastfeeding working mother.

TELL YOUR EMPLOYER!

Supporting you to continue nursing is in your employer's interests. Breastfeeding means your baby will continue to receive his daily update of live antibodies (see page 5), which will reduce the chances of his becoming sick and requiring you to take time off work to look after him. Breastfeeding also boosts *your* immunity and helps regulate your metabolism, so you are less likely to be sick, too.

KEY POINTS

- You can keep breastfeeding going, even if you can't be with your baby all the time.
- If you have to be apart from your baby, you can express and store your milk for him.
- You can express your milk by hand or with a pump—or use a combination of both.
- When you first start expressing, you may not get much milk. If you concentrate on putting in the order, your production will soon increase.

- Think about your own need to express as well as your baby's need for milk, when planning how you will manage separations.
- If you have to be apart from your baby, aim to breastfeed as often as possible when you're with him, to allow him to catch up and to help maintain your milk production.
- Your baby may not need to use a bottle; if he is four months or older when you have to leave him, he may prefer an open cup or sippy cup.
- Lots of babies refuse to take expressed breastmilk or formula. They don't starve—they just make up for it with lots of feedings later.
- Discussing your child's feeding with his caretaker in advance is an important part of minimizing disruption to breastfeeding.
- If you are going back to work, tell your employer in advance you are planning to continue breastfeeding. Employers are legally obliged to allow you breaks so that you can express your milk in a clean, private area.

10

Six Months and Beyond

BREAST MILK IS all your baby needs for the first six months of her life, and you can expect it to remain her main source of nourishment until she is around a year old. However, from the middle of her first year, she'll start to move toward solid foods and family mealtimes. These will gradually take over until, eventually, she stops having breast milk feedings altogether. This transition is called weaning, and when baby-led, it usually takes *at least* a year. If you keep following your baby's instincts, the move to family meals will go at a pace that is naturally right for her, allowing her to continue having as much milk as she needs alongside as much (or as little) solid food as she wants. This is known as baby-led weaning.

Like baby-led breastfeeding, baby-led weaning relies on your baby's natural instincts and abilities to begin eating solid foods when she is ready. It's very different from the parent-led, stage-by-stage, conventional approach to introducing solids. It's a combination of:

- sharing mealtimes with your baby
- allowing her to set the pace
- trusting her to know what she needs
- trusting her to feed herself

This chapter explains how baby-led weaning works and how you can give your baby the opportunity to include solid foods in her diet when she is ready. It also looks at how you can continue to let her lead the way with nursing as she gets older, so that her last breastfeeding happens at a time that is right for her.

Starting Solid Foods the Baby-Led Way

Learning to eat solid food is a natural and inevitable part of development for any healthy baby—just like crawling, walking, and talking. And, like those activities, if it's allowed to, it will begin spontaneously, at the right time for each baby.

Most babies' digestive and immune systems are not able to cope with anything other than breast milk or formula before about six months. If they are given other foods earlier than this, they may not be able to digest them fully—and, if they are breastfed, they will tend to take less milk to make room for them. This is why nowadays, solid foods are not recommended before six months. If your four-month-old really *is* hungry, she will get more nourishment from nursing more often than she will from other foods.

The skills and coordination your baby needs for handling food develop at about the same rate as her need for a more varied diet and the ability of her gut to digest other foods. The traditional signs of readiness for solids that parents have been told to look out for, such as waking at night and watching other people eating, are now known to have nothing to do with needing other foods. They are simply a normal part of a baby's development that start to happen at around four months old. You will know your baby is truly ready when she can sit upright, reach out and grab objects, take them to her mouth, and gnaw on them with her gums. In other words, if you give her the opportunity, she will start by herself.

Of course, babies develop at different rates, so some will be reaching for food a week or so before six months while for others it will be several weeks later. For a rough summary, see "What to Expect When," page 280. The important thing, in a baby-led approach to introducing solids, is that it should be *your baby's* decision to reach for food, and her decision to take it to her mouth.

NO NEED FOR ONE FOOD AT A TIME

If you have waited until your baby is truly ready for solid foods, there is no need to follow the cautious "one new food at a time" rule that you may have been told about. This is because you can be confident that your baby's gut is ready to digest a wider range of foods. The only exception is when there are allergies in the family, in which case the one-at-a-time rule is preferable for foods that may produce an allergic reaction.

Why Self-Feeding Makes Sense

By the time your baby is ready to start discovering how to eat solid foods, she has already developed most of the skills she needs to do it. She has been feeding herself (as opposed to "being fed") since her very first breastfeeding (see Chapter 4), and because of the way she's used her mouth muscles, she's strengthened them for chewing. She's also been watching you eat and practicing picking things up and taking them to her mouth. And she's been tasting your food through your milk.

Because of this, most babies instinctively want—and are able—to figure out how to feed themselves with their fingers. There's no need for spoon feeding. And because by six months they can chew most foods (whether or not they have teeth), there's no need for their food to be pureed. Spoon feeding is appropriate for babies who are not able to feed themselves (those with certain physical disabilities or delayed development, for example) but the vast majority of six-month-olds don't need it.

Breastfed babies are used to controlling how much they eat and how quickly, and whether to have just a drink or a full, fat-rich feeding (see page 28), and they can continue to make these decisions when they move on to solid foods. **Allowing babies to feed themselves ensures they eat what they need and don't cut down on breast milk before they're ready.** It also enables them to learn how to manage different textures confidently and safely. Recent research shows that babies who were introduced to solid foods this way make healthier food choices and may be less prone to obesity in later childhood.

> "From the beginning, I nursed Mia whenever she wanted. Sometimes, she wouldn't have much, and other times, she seemed to gorge herself. When it came to solids, of course, she had to stay in control—it seemed insane to suddenly start stuffing her full of mush just to make *me* feel better. She eats really well and has however much she needs, just as she always has done. There's no stress at mealtimes; we just sit and eat together. It's great."
>
> Kirsty, mother of Mia, 2 years

Will My Baby Eat Enough Food?

Most babies don't actually *eat* any solid food for several weeks after they start handling it. This is normal; they need to learn about tastes and textures, and to practice chewing, before they start to rely on food for nourishment. In a healthy, full-term baby, the combination of breast milk and the nutrients stored in her body while she was in the womb are enough to ensure full nutrition until she's *at least* six months old—and probably until she is eight or nine months.

From six months onward, your baby will begin to need very small amounts of additional nutrients (mainly iron and zinc), which she will get by gradually expanding her diet—but she won't need to eat large quantities; small tastes will be enough. The first sign that she has managed to swallow something will probably be when you see tiny pieces of it in her poop, but she will continue to have "breastfeeding poop" (runny and yellow), with occasional bits, for several months after she has started exploring other foods. Later, as she begins to eat more, her stools will start to become more solid, darker, and smellier—especially once she starts to cut down her intake of breast milk.

At some point—often around eight or nine months—babies seem to make the connection between hunger and solid food. It's then that they begin to eat more purposefully, as though they are actually hungry, and to play with food less. It's likely that this coincides with their growing need for extra nutrition.

Provided your baby has been allowed to handle food as often as she wants, by the time she needs additional nutrients she will be an accomplished eater and able to manage a wide variety of foods, so she will have no problem getting them.

Breastfeeding alongside the introduction of solid foods not only ensures good nutrition, it actually helps with the digestion of those other foods. It's thought the unique ingredients of human milk may also reduce the chances of food allergies and intolerances, such as celiac disease. Infant formula and "toddler" or Step 2 formulas cannot provide this sort of protection.

Coming to Grips with Solid Foods

If your baby is given the opportunity to show you when she is ready to begin handling food, she will simply grab some from the table, take it to her mouth, and start munching on it. At first she'll have most success with larger pieces of food that she can pick up easily, with some sticking out of her fist. As she becomes more dexterous she'll learn to manage smaller pieces (and eventually progress to using cutlery).

Your baby's motivation to try solid foods is not hunger. After all, she doesn't yet know that food can fill her tummy. She is driven by curiosity and her instinct to develop new skills. She will experiment with food just as she does with a new toy, exploring it with her hands and her mouth, squishing, smearing, and licking it and discovering what it can do. Gradually, she'll learn to bite off pieces with her gums and figure out how to chew them. The first few times she does this, as long as she is sitting upright, the food will fall out of her mouth. Then, when she has developed the ability to move chewed food to the back of her mouth, some will be swallowed.

It's better, in the early days, if your baby *isn't* hungry when you offer her the chance to handle food. If she is, she'll get frustrated— just as she would if you tried to interest her in a new toy when all she wanted was to nurse. Mealtimes are playtimes in the beginning; if your baby is hungry or thirsty, it's your breast she needs.

What Happens with Breastfeeding?

For the first few months after she starts solid food, anything your baby eats will be *in addition to* her milk, and breastfeeding will carry on much as before. Then, sometime around nine months, she'll begin gradually to need less breast milk. However, unless she is having other drinks (which would decrease her need for breast milk as a drink), the number of breastfeedings she asks for probably won't change noticeably at first; she will simply carry on asking to nurse in her usual way but take slightly less milk. In time, you'll notice that she asks for some milk feedings a little later than usual, especially after a meal where she's eaten quite a lot of solid food.

Then, when she is regularly eating and drinking at mealtimes, she may decide to skip some breastfeedings altogether, turning away when she's offered the breast. All you need to do is to respond to her cues, just as you have until now.

Even if you notice a fairly consistent drop in breastfeeding, it may not be a permanent change. It's common for babies to go back to nursing more often and lose interest in solid foods for short periods, especially when they are teething or fighting off an infection. They may want nothing but breast milk for a week or two, then switch back to eating solid foods and taking less milk. Babies also tend to want to breastfeed more often when they are feeling emotionally unsettled. If you go back to work (see page 161), move, or go on vacation, for instance, you can expect your baby to ask to nurse more often to help her cope with the change, whether or not she is eating much solid food.

If your baby's appetite for milk lessens but then suddenly increases again, your breasts will start to adapt immediately—even if your milk production has already gone down considerably. If you let her feed as much as she wants, your supply will soon catch up.

Babies rarely stop breastfeeding of their own accord before their first birthday. If your baby is under a year old and turns down the offer of a breastfeeding several times in a row, don't assume she's ready to give up the breast. It's more likely she's going through a nursing strike (see page 129). She'll probably go back to breastfeeding within a few days if you continue to offer her the opportunity.

BABY-LED WEANING AT A GLANCE

HOW TO START:

- As soon as your baby can sit up with little or no support, start including her in your mealtimes and snacks whenever possible. Choose times when she is not hungry or sleepy.
- Make sure the food you are eating is healthy, so your baby can share it and copy you as you eat.
- Prepare for some mess. Lots of food will go on the floor to start with. A clean splash mat under the chair means you can reoffer food that has been dropped. A plate is not necessary at first and may be a distraction.
- Sit your baby on your lap or in a highchair. Make sure she is sitting upright and that she can reach the table or tray easily.
- Let her share the food on your plate, or put a few pieces of food in front of her for her to pick up (babies can be overwhelmed by too much choice).
- Offer your baby water to drink with her meals—but don't be surprised if she isn't interested. She may prefer to continue to have all her drinks at the breast.
- Continue to offer the breast whenever she asks for it.

FOODS TO OFFER:

- Prepare nutritious food so that your baby can pick it up easily— thick sticks of vegetables (2 to 3 ½ inches long), pieces of fruit, strips of meat, and fingers of toast are all suitable to start with.
- Include new shapes and textures gradually so that your baby has the chance to practice and develop her skills. Rice, ground or chopped meat, and runny, crunchy, or slippery foods all provide interesting challenges.

- Aim for a variety of flavors. Babies don't need bland food (many strong flavors will be familiar to her from your breast milk). Unless there are allergies in your family, there is no need to start with one taste at a time.
- Avoid salt, sugar, additives, prepackaged meals, and other foods that are unsuitable for babies, such as honey, under-cooked eggs, and peanuts.

WHAT TO EXPECT:

- Mealtimes are for learning and experimenting, at first, so your baby probably won't eat much for the first few months. Provided she can breastfeed whenever she wants, breast milk will continue to provide all her nourishment.
- Many babies gag on food in the early weeks. This is a normal protective reflex to push food forward, away from the airway, while they are learning how to manage it. The gag reflex is more sensitive in babies than adults and is triggered farther forward on the tongue. It's *not* the same as choking and it doesn't seem to bother babies. Once the food has been pushed forward, either it falls out of their mouth or they carry on chewing it.

REMEMBER TO:

- Keep mealtimes enjoyable—let your baby play, and don't hurry her or try to persuade her to eat more than she wants.
- Trust your baby to cut down her milk feedings whenever she is ready.
- Explain how baby-led weaning works to anyone involved in feeding your baby.

(Continued on next page)

SAFETY:

- Make sure your baby is sitting upright to eat, not leaning back in a bouncy chair or slumping forward or sideways. This will allow her to control the food in her mouth safely.
- Don't put anything in your baby's mouth for her—and don't let anyone else do so, either (watch out for "helpful" toddlers).
- Don't offer your baby hard nuts (in pieces or whole); remove pits from food such as olives and cherries; cut small, round fruits, such as grapes, in half.
- Never leave your baby alone with food.

    See "Sources of Information and Support," page 293, for where to get more information on baby-led weaning.

Breastfeeding as Your Child Grows Older

Breastfeeding doesn't have to end just because your baby is no longer relying on it for her nourishment—it can continue for several more years, if you both want. The World Health Organization recommends that all babies should be breastfed for at least two years (with complementary foods from six months), but there isn't an upper age limit. Many young children continue to nurse two or three times a day—perhaps first thing in the morning and last thing at night, plus random times when they fall over or are tired or upset—well into early childhood. And continuing to breastfeed will benefit *your* health, too (see page 6).

Many women expect to stop breastfeeding by the time their child reaches a certain age. Sometimes this is because they are unaware that it's normal for children to continue to breastfeed into their second, third, or fourth year—perhaps because nursing at this age usually happens at home and is rarely talked about. However, many of those who had planned to stop breastfeeding after, for instance, a year or eighteen months, find, when the time comes, that they no longer want to stop. If both you and your child are enjoying this special time together, there's no need for it to end. Stopping before one of you is ready can be challenging (see "Ending Breastfeeding—Who Decides?," page 182); it's easier to continue until the time feels right for you both.

> "I haven't made a decision to carry on breastfeeding Celia—but the decision to stop will be hers. Sometimes I've thought I'll stop soon but it's never felt right just to take it away from her. At night she has a couple of sucks to get to sleep. In the morning, we'll spend a good hour feeding if we have the time. It's becoming gradually less and less. A year ago there's no way she would have said no if I offered her the chance to nurse, but now she says no sometimes. She'll stop when she's ready—I'm in no hurry."
> Miranda, mother of Celia, 2 years

Many people assume that, once a baby is having a good, varied diet of solid foods, there's no value in breast milk. This isn't true. **The protective factors in your milk will continue to help your child resist infections for as long as you continue to feed her.** As she starts to drink less and your production winds down, your milk will become gradually more concentrated—almost like colostrum again—giving her an extra boost of immunity as she faces the rough and tumble of childhood. In fact, a child's immune system is not fully mature until she is about six years old, so it's reasonable to assume that children can continue to benefit from the antibodies in breast milk until they are well past toddlerhood.

Breast milk doesn't lose its nutritional properties just because the child is eating other foods. It continues to provide balanced nutrition and is the single most complete food available to humans. Research has shown that children who stop breastfeeding before two years of age have a greater risk of illness and take longer to recover than those who nurse for longer. Continuing to breastfeed means you will always have a nourishing, easy-to-digest food to give your child if she becomes sick, and many mothers keep nursing through the toddler years for this reason alone.

However, feeding a toddler is very different from feeding a newborn, so you may need to make some adjustments to the way breastfeeding happens to enable you and your child to continue enjoying this part of your relationship.

Toddlers Aren't Always Discreet!

By the time your baby reaches her first birthday, she'll be very quick and efficient at breastfeeding and able to latch on from virtually any angle. However, as she grows in confidence and dexterity, you may find that she asks for feedings in ways that you don't really like.

Toddlers want to exert their independence and show everyone what they can do. They don't understand that their mother may not want them to start helping themselves to her breast—by pulling up her top and grabbing at her bra—when they are in a café or at the mall. So you may want to give your child some guidance on how you'd like her to behave when she wants to nurse.

Many mothers have a word for breastfeeding that they use from very early on when they offer their baby a feeding—"booby" or "mommy milk," for example. If you are likely to be embarrassed when your baby learns to talk and starts asking for "booby," you may want to opt for a more neutral word from the outset. You can then encourage her to ask for a feeding quietly, using her special word, rather than announcing her intentions loudly (or just helping herself). Some women choose a word that won't mean anything to anyone else (except perhaps another breastfeeding mother)— "noo-noo," for example. Others use a phrase such as "mommy hug" or "sleepy hug," which won't raise any eyebrows.

As she gets older, your child will begin to be able to wait a little while to nurse. This will be useful if you are in a place where you don't feel comfortable feeding her. You'll find you can distract her so that she forgets for a while, or if she's old enough, simply tell her, when she asks, that she can have milk later.

Dealing with Negative Opinions

Many people don't know about the benefits of breastfeeding past babyhood and they may feel uncomfortable about toddlers and young children being breastfed. For the generation of parents (now grandparents and great-grandparents) who were encouraged to get their child to do everything early (solids by three months, no milk feedings past a year, and so on) it can be especially puzzling.

You will probably find it useful to have a few strategies to help you deal with awkward questions and unsupportive comments. For example, you could explain the reasons that breastfeeding is beneficial for small children. Or you may prefer to say that health professionals advise breastfeeding for as long as possible. Alternatively, you could simply decide that you don't need to justify your breastfeeding relationship with your child to anyone, and change the subject.

You may find it helpful to make contact with other mothers who are breastfeeding older babies and children, perhaps through a group such as La Leche League (see "Sources of Information and Support," page 290).

Breastfeeding During Pregnancy and Beyond

Many women become pregnant while they are still breastfeeding an older child (although, when breastfeeding is baby led, it's unusual for a mother to become pregnant again within six months—see page 142), and there is rarely a reason that it is not safe for them to continue. Women who are prone to miscarriage or premature birth are occasionally advised to stop breastfeeding for part of their pregnancy, but in general, a mother's body is perfectly able to nourish two babies at the same time.

Breastfeeding When You're Pregnant

Some mothers find that breastfeeding continues smoothly throughout their next pregnancy, but most notice changes as their body prepares for a new arrival. Mother and baby can usually find ways of adapting their technique to accommodate what is happening, but occasionally the changes mean that nursing has to end early.

The most obvious cause of disruption to breastfeeding is the growing bump. This may make some of your usual nursing positions uncomfortable or impossible. If you can, explain to your child that your tummy is tender and enlist her help to find a position that works for both of you.

Another common problem is increased tenderness of the nipples, which can make breastfeeding painful—either for a few weeks or, in some cases, for most of the pregnancy. Negotiating shorter feedings with your child, and making sure she doesn't "play" with your other nipple or keep coming on and off the breast may make feeding more tolerable.

The other key change is to the breast milk itself. Although some women carry on making large quantities of milk throughout their pregnancy, most find that their breasts revert to producing colostrum, ready for the new baby. This changes the taste and consistency of the milk, and the amount available—which is likely to be noticed by the breastfeeding child. A simple explanation may be enough to help your child cope with this development, but she may decide that she prefers not to nurse, at least temporarily.

Some toddlers decide to wean themselves off the breast while their mother is pregnant and then want to start nursing again when the new baby arrives. If you are prepared for this to happen, and welcome it, your child is less likely to feel rejected in favor of the new arrival.

> "When I was pregnant with Charlie, my breasts were so tender I had to clamp my jaws together whenever Grace fed. But I wanted her to decide when she was ready to stop and I wanted her and the new baby to feed together. Then one night she latched on and said: 'Mommy, no milk.' I don't know if there wasn't any or she didn't want any. I was relieved in a way, but also sad that I wouldn't be tandem nursing. But a few months after Charlie was born, she asked to try it again, so I did it after all."
>
> Jade, mother of Grace, 2 years,
> and Charlie, 9 months

Whether or not your toddler is still breastfeeding near the end of your pregnancy, she won't have forgotten about it. However, she won't automatically know that new babies need to do it, so if she's old enough to understand, it's important to explain this to her. It may help to show her pictures of herself as a baby, and to point out that newborns can't eat all the other sorts of food that she enjoys, which means they need to drink lots of breast milk. Taking her to visit a friend who is nursing a young baby (or to a breastfeeding support group) may help her understand that new babies need to breastfeed often, rather than just occasionally.

You Can Breastfeed Your Baby and Your Older Child

Breastfeeding siblings who are different in age (or "tandem" nursing) can be one of the best ways of preventing an older brother or sister from feeling rejected or jealous of a new baby. For many women it happens naturally, especially if there's not much gap between their pregnancies, while others plan to tandem nurse specifically to ease the transition for their older child. However, some negotiation may be necessary to ensure that the new baby gets what she needs.

In the first few days, if your older child wants to feed at around the same time as her new sibling, it's best to ask her to wait, just to be sure the new baby gets her share of colostrum. The exception to this is if you are still producing large volumes of milk; in this case, allowing your toddler to feed first will help lessen the flow and make it easier for your new baby to manage. **Including both baby and child in breastfeeding will encourage your milk production to increase rapidly, so there will soon be plenty for two.** (Expect your toddler to have a brief bout of loose stools, brought on by drinking colostrum.)

Holding a toddler and a new baby so they can nurse at the same time can present a challenge. In the first few weeks, the easiest way for you to feed your children together may be lying back on your bed, with your new baby on top of you and your toddler next to you. If you prefer to sit up, try asking your toddler to sit or kneel (or stand) beside you to nurse, to give you more room to position your little one.

If you are used to your toddler pretty much helping herself at the breast, you may be surprised to rediscover how much support your newborn needs and how long it takes her to feed. Giving your new baby the time she needs to figure out how to latch on while you have an older child wanting to share you may not be easy. Some mothers enlist their older child's help to show her sibling what to do, while others insist that the new baby be allowed to nurse separately or to get started first, before the toddler joins in.

It's common for older children to want to negotiate which breast is "theirs." While it will usually be possible to nurse your new baby exclusively from the breast that her sibling has allocated to her, if she is taking a while to get the hang of breastfeeding you may have to ask your older child to feed from that breast, too, to ensure both breasts are "asked" to make plenty of milk.

Toddlers can be unpredictable about how often they want to breastfeed. For the first few weeks after the baby's birth, while your milk production is unsettled, your breasts may become overfull at times, making it difficult for your newborn to attach and putting you at risk of engorgement or mastitis. Encouraging some consistency in your toddler's nursing pattern will help keep things on an even keel. Of course, if your breasts do become uncomfortable, your older child is the ideal person to help relieve them.

Tandem nursing, even when planned, can sometimes be difficult emotionally for the mother, especially in the first week or so. You may be surprised to find your protective instincts for your newborn kicking in suddenly, so much so that you even feel resentful toward your older child when she wants to nurse. This is entirely normal and is nature's way of ensuring that the most vulnerable member of the family is cared for. But it may mean that the transition to tandem nursing isn't quite as seamless as you'd envisioned. And if these emotions coincide with your older child feeling left out and demanding more of your attention, life could become stressful. Sharing your feelings with your partner or with another mother who has tandem nursed may help (if you don't know anyone to talk to, you may find an online forum or the La Leche League helpline useful—see "Sources of Information and Support," page 290). Having special time alone with each child, and remembering how much your older child may need the emotional reassurance of breastfeeding at this time, can also help.

"Tandem nursing was hard at first. The new baby latching on was like learning how to breastfeed all over again and Micky wanted milk at the same time. Sometimes it would be easier to feed Micky first. Toddlers often need just a little to be satisfied—it's more about comfort and knowing they can still have the breast, and he was so needy because of the new baby."

Sharon, mother of Micky, 4 years,
and Carly, 2 years

If one of your children is sick, both you and the other child will already have been exposed to any germs, so you needn't change the way you feed them. If the older one has an infection, the antibodies in your milk will help prevent your newborn from becoming sick—or help her recover quickly—and will also help your toddler get well faster. The only exception to this is if either child gets an infection of the mouth (such as thrush; see page 240). In that case, if you spot the problem early, allocating them one breast each may help prevent the other child (and breast) from developing the condition—although you should still get treatment for both breasts and both children, just to be sure.

Ending Breastfeeding—Who Decides?

In many cases breastfeeding ends naturally, as the child outgrows her need for it. In others, the mother makes the decision to stop. However, it's rare for babies who've been allowed to set the pace with weaning to be ready to manage without milk feedings before they are at least a year old. **If you have to (or choose to) stop breastfeeding when your baby is under 12 months, you'll need to give her formula.** See page 230 for how to replace breastfeeding with formula, and for what to do if you need or want to stop breastfeeding quickly.

When the end of breastfeeding is chosen by the child, it can be either quite sudden or a gradual process. Some children announce that they don't want to nurse anymore; others continue to have one feeding a day until something, such as a holiday, changes the usual routine and the breast gets forgotten. Even when it seems as though your toddler has had her last breastfeeding, she may surprise you by asking to nurse again two weeks later.

Breastfeeding doesn't always end at a time that both mother and child are happy with. Sometimes, the mother is ready to stop before her child has gotten to that point; in other cases, it's the mother who finds it difficult to accept her child's decision to stop. If you and your child (over a year old) aren't ready for nursing to end at the same time, you may find the following suggestions helpful for working things out.

FEELING UNDER PRESSURE TO STOP

Sometimes mothers feel under pressure from their partners, family, or friends to stop breastfeeding. But giving up something you're enjoying may be very hard emotionally—for you and your child. Stopping when neither of you is truly ready may make family life miserable and could lead to resentment.

What If I Want to Stop but My Child Doesn't?

Some mothers want to stop nursing because they "want their body back" or because a new chapter is opening in their life—a new pregnancy, for example, or a new job. Although breastfeeding does not have to end in these circumstances, you may choose to leave it behind as part of this transition.

If you are simply fed up with your child asking for milk at

awkward times, all you might need to do is to cut back her nursing gradually (see page 230), until she is having only a couple of feedings a day—maybe bedtime and morning—then reassess how you feel. It may be that you simply need to be feeding less, rather than not at all.

If you *do* want to stop but your child wants to continue, be prepared for the process to take several weeks. She needs time to come to terms with what is happening, and your breasts need time to decrease production gradually. Try to avoid periods that are likely to be emotionally unsettling for her, such as around her starting preschool or the arrival of a new baby, and be ready to put things on hold if she is upset or sick. Remember that even if breastfeeding is driving *you* crazy, your child may still love it and feel rejected and confused when you want to take it away.

Helping Your Child Give Up the Breast

There are several strategies you can choose from to bring about the end of breastfeeding for a baby over a year old:

- *Don't offer, don't refuse.* Rather than offer feedings when your child would normally want them, simply wait for her to ask. If it turns out that she was ready to stop nursing anyway, this method may be very quick, in which case you may find yourself offering the occasional feeding after all so that you don't have to express to stay comfortable.

- *Distraction.* When you sense that your child is about to ask to nurse, suggest a distraction, such as a game or a trip to the playground. This can work very well for daytime feedings, especially at a time when there are lots of exciting activities, such as when you are on vacation. Distracting your child *before* she asks to nurse, rather than trying to divert her when she has already decided that's what she needs, will prevent her becoming upset.

- *Make yourself unavailable.* Get your partner or someone else to take over your child's care at key times—such as bedtime—for a while. If necessary, arrange to be out of the house (perhaps by inventing an urgent errand). Make sure she is still having plenty of hugs and affection from you at other times. If she usually breast-feeds to help her doze off for a nap, a drive in the car or (if she is still small enough) a walk in the stroller or sling may work instead.

- *Negotiate a date with your child* (for instance, her next birthday, July 4th, or the first/last day of an exciting holiday), then cut out feedings gradually, working toward that date. This can work well with an older child, who is able to understand the concept of time. Don't insist on the earliest possible date—it's impor-tant that your child feels she's agreed to the plan. Be prepared to renegotiate if she changes her mind when the time comes.

- *Planned schedule.* This approach only really works if your child's breastfeeding pattern is fairly consistent from day to day. Just cut out one feeding at a time, allowing a few days in between for your breasts to adjust. To minimize discomfort, try to keep the gaps between remaining feedings as even as possible. Expect her to resist losing the last feeding more strongly than she does the others.

Whichever approach you choose, make sure you have plenty of healthy snacks and drinks on hand for times when your child is likely to be hungry or thirsty. You may also find it helpful to mini-mize reminders that could trigger a request to nurse; for example, by opting for a trip to the park when you'd normally be nursing on the couch, wearing perfume to mask the smell of your milk, not letting your child see your naked breasts, and choosing tops without easy access to them.

Nighttime feedings are likely to be the last to go, and they can be the hardest to stop. Making your breasts less available at night—for example, by wearing a high-necked T-shirt—and having some water or expressed breast milk to offer your child if she wakes can help. Alternatively, your partner can cuddle with your child at bedtime, or rock her to sleep, and be the person who sleeps nearest to her at night to comfort her if she wakes. If your child is old enough to understand, encouraging her to say good night at bedtime to all the different things that have to go to sleep at night: the birds, the sun, her friends—and your breasts, will (eventually) mean she doesn't expect them to be available if she wakes. However, it's rare that stopping nursing at night means that a child stops waking during the night altogether; you may find it takes you slightly longer to comfort your child when that happens, without breastfeeding to soothe her back to sleep. Some mothers are happy to keep nursing at night long after daytime feedings have stopped, for this reason.

"I had to stop feeding Ryan when he was two for medical reasons. It was hard. Feedings during the day went first, because he was easily distracted. But every morning he'd wake up and say, 'Milk, Mommy,' and he'd feed. Then, eventually one morning he said, 'Cereal.' The night feed went after that—I told him to say good-bye to nursing and his dad put him to bed. The whole thing took several months. With Jamie, my youngest, I wanted him to nurse for as long as possible, but he decided himself just before his third birthday. He just came off the breast, looked at it, and walked away. I knew then that it was his last feeding. There was no real warning—I was devastated."

Natalie, mother of Ryan, 6 years,
and Jamie, 3 years

What If My Child Wants to Stop but I Don't?

Sometimes women find their child has had enough of the breast long before they expected them to. If you have read all about the nutritional, immunological, and emotional benefits of feeding a child for several years but your toddler decides she can do without it, this can be bitterly disappointing. Many mothers mourn the passing of the special closeness of their breastfeeding relationship, especially if it has ended suddenly.

It's impossible to persuade a child to breastfeed when she doesn't want to because *she* has to do the feeding—all you do is provide the breast. So if your child decides to stop nursing, there will probably be little you can do to change her mind. However, the following may be worth a try:

- If your child uses a pacifier or has a bottle, these may be satisfying her need to suck; discouraging their use may tempt her back to the breast.
- Continuing to offer her the chance to nurse at times when she used to particularly enjoy it, such as at bedtime, or when she is tired or upset, may rekindle her interest.
- Some of the suggestions for overcoming a nursing strike (see page 130), such as sharing a bath with your child, may remind her what she is missing.

Generally, be available for her, but don't nag her to breastfeed—it's unlikely to win her over. If you feel your child has stopped breastfeeding before you would have liked, it may help to remind yourself that baby-led breastfeeding is about trusting your child's decisions throughout—including her ability to know when her need for breastfeeding is over. She is still young and will continue to need plenty of mommy time.

KEY POINTS

- At around six months, your baby is likely to be ready to begin experimenting with solid foods. Her natural instincts and abilities will make it easy for her to feed herself.

- If you offer your baby the chance to join in with healthy family meals, she will show you when she is ready to share your food.

- If your baby is allowed to decide how much solid food to eat, she will cut down her milk feedings gradually, at a pace that is right for her.

- Breastfeeding beyond one year is normal and natural— babies under a year old are very unlikely to stop breast-feeding of their own accord.

- Many children continue nursing once or twice a day for several years. Breast milk never loses its protective proper-ties, and breastfeeding is one of the best ways to comfort a young child.

- You may want to figure out with your toddler some dis-creet ways for her to ask to nurse.

- If you want to, you can continue to breastfeed when you are pregnant—and continue nursing your older child when the new baby arrives.

- Ideally, breastfeeding will come to a natural conclusion when you and your child are both ready. If it has to happen earlier than this, there are strategies you can employ to help you both make the adjustment.

Part III

Less Common Situations

11

Premature Babies and Multiples

BABIES OFTEN COME early, and they sometimes come in pairs, threes, or more. Having a baby born prematurely or having more than one baby (whether or not they are born early) brings all sorts of challenges for parents, but it doesn't mean breastfeeding isn't possible or that it can't be at least partly baby led. This chapter looks at how to recognize your baby's (or babies') abilities and make the most of them so that together you can benefit from the unique start that breastfeeding brings.

Breastfeeding When Your Baby Is Born Early

When a baby is born early, all previous plans go out the window. Nothing quite prepares you for the shock of becoming a parent earlier than you originally anticipated. The support of people who understand what you're going through can be invaluable. (See "Sources of Information and Support," page 292, for a useful website.)

Your little one will probably need to be cared for in a neonatal intensive care unit (NICU). Depending on how premature he is, he may have wires attached to him to monitor his heart rate and oxygen levels, he may have an intravenous line in place and a tube through his nose or mouth into his stomach, and he may need help to breathe. And, of course, since premature births are often accompanied by illness in the mother and/or by some sort of instrumental delivery, you may not be fully well or mobile yourself.

Why Breast Milk Is Important for Premature Babies

Breast milk is even more important for your baby if he is born prematurely than it would be if he had arrived on time. This is because his gut is more immature (and less able to tolerate formula milk) and his vulnerability to infection even greater than if he had stayed a bit longer in the womb. In fact, breast milk is so important for a premature baby's health, both immediately and long term, that many on the staff of NICUs think of breast milk as primarily a medicine rather than as a food.

Donor human milk can be obtained from a breast milk bank, but whenever possible, the ideal milk for a premature baby is his own mother's milk, and especially her colostrum. The best thing you can do for your newborn premature baby is to provide him with your milk from the very beginning.

However, a premature birth presents several challenges in terms of getting breastfeeding up and running, and you'll find you are faced with two main obstacles:

- You and your baby are likely to be separated. This may be only briefly or it may be for long periods of time, perhaps extending over several months. Skin-to-skin contact may not be possible for hours, days, or even weeks after the birth. And if your baby has to stay in the hospital, privacy will be hard to come by.
- Your baby may be too weak or immature to breastfeed, at first.

Expressing Milk for Your Premature Baby

If your baby is premature, he may not be able to breastfeed right away and may not even be ready for milk feedings. But although he'll be getting all his nourishment intravenously, he will still benefit from your colostrum. A few drops spread around the inside of his mouth will help protect him from infections, start to strengthen his digestive tract, and help him recognize your taste and smell. You can provide your milk for him—by expressing—as soon as he's born. (You'll find information on expressing breast milk on page 86 and in Chapter 9.)

Expressing your milk as soon as possible after the birth is also enormously important to set up your breasts for long-term milk production. When a baby is born on time, the messages the breasts receive during the first two weeks (and especially the first few days) are what determine how much milk the mother is able to make in the future (see Chapter 2). But when a baby arrives early, much of what would normally happen to trigger milk production isn't possible. So to ensure plenty of milk, both now and later, you'll need to mimic the frequent nursing your baby would have done if he'd been born closer to his due date.

The key to getting milk production going by expressing is to start early and do it often. If you can express intensively over the first two weeks (see page 195), you'll give your breasts a huge "wake-up call," and your chances of being able to breastfeed your baby for as long as you want will be vastly increased. Your breasts will need this extra stimulation even if your baby is managing to have some of his feedings at the breast, because he won't have the strength or the appetite to put in a big enough order on his own. Make sure your partner and family understand how important this time is, so they can give you the support you need to focus on expressing.

Because of the intensive nature of expressing for a premature baby, the hospital staff should make sure you have access to an electric breast pump while you're there. You may be able to rent a pump directly from them or from a commercial company by searching online to find your nearest pump rental station. Many mothers find a pump very useful after the first few days. However, colostrum comes in very small amounts and is quite sticky, so hand expression (see page 86) is a much better way to collect this first milk. If someone can sit with you and draw it up in a little syringe as you express it, your baby will be sure to get every drop.

"Frankie was seven weeks premature and was in an incubator for two weeks. It was really hard to express at first—it felt like there was nothing there. They showed me how to hand express, so I had milk ready for him once he was off the intravenous line. I used to set my alarm so I could do it every three hours, day and night. After ten days I started feeding him myself, but it took him about two weeks to open his mouth properly—he used to suck as if my breast was a straw. I was in agony—every night I'd swear I'd give up—then in the morning I'd change my mind. I nursed him until he was 10 months but now I wish I'd done it for longer."

Kerry, mother of Ella, 8; Joshua, 6; and Frankie, 14 months

The NICU staff will be able to guide you on how to store your milk, and some NICUs will provide you with containers and labels. All the equipment needs to be sterile because premature babies are especially vulnerable to infection. Ideally, your baby should have your milk as soon as possible after you've expressed it; if it needs to be refrigerated or frozen, it should be given to him in the order it was expressed—at least in the first couple of weeks—so you'll need to label each batch clearly with the time you expressed it as well as the date. (Where possible, fresh milk is always preferable to refrigerated or frozen milk because some of the protective ingredients are deactivated by cold.)

How to Give Your Breasts a Two-Week "Wake-Up Call" If
Your Baby Is Premature or Sick

The more you stimulate your breasts to make milk in the first
two weeks, the easier breastfeeding will be from then on. It's also
important to build up a store of milk in case you experience a dip
in supply later (see tip on page 197). Here's what to do:

- If you and your baby are well enough, spend as long as you
  can immediately after the birth with him lying against
  your tummy and chest, skin to skin. Hold him like this as
  often as possible over the next few weeks.
- Start expressing as soon as you can after your baby is
  born—within an hour is good. If you don't feel well
  enough to do it yourself, ask your partner or a midwife to
  do it for you. Hand expressing is best at this stage.
- **Express as often as you can, day and night. Aim for
  twelve times in twenty-four hours**—certainly no fewer
  than eight. The intervals between sessions don't need to be
  regular—just fit them in whenever you can.
- Try to avoid long gaps—four hours during the day (or six
  hours at night) should be the absolute maximum. Plan
  ahead: If you know you're going to need a gap of more than
  two or three hours, see whether you can fit in some extra
  expressing before and afterward. If you are in a place where
  you can't save the milk, express anyway and throw it away.
  You'll have more milk in the long run if you keep putting in
  the order.
- Use some of the tips on page 152 to get your oxytocin
  flowing before and during each expressing session. If
  you can't be near your baby, close your eyes and visualize
  yourself holding him, stroking him, smelling him, and

kissing him. Try to include a few minutes of breast massage at every session. If you can be with your baby but can't hold him, ask the NICU staff to help you to get some privacy near him for expressing—for instance by putting a screen around you both—to make it easier to get your milk flowing.

- Hand express or use a pump, whichever you prefer. Ideally, express by hand while the amounts are small and move on to a combination of hand and pump as the volume increases, starting and finishing each session with hand expression.

- If you're using a pump, make sure the flange (or funnel) is the right size for you so that it compresses your milk ducts effectively. Ask the staff for help with this, and don't be afraid to experiment with larger or smaller flanges to find the one that suits you.

- Start each pumping session with the pump on a low setting and increase the rate and strength gradually, as the milk starts to flow. There is no need to aim for maximum power; just find the level that works best for you.

- When the milk stops flowing with a pump, do a bit of breast massage and then some hand expression. This will usually trigger another let-down reflex. Then go back to the pump. When the flow subsides again, wait a couple of minutes and have another go. You'll be surprised how much extra milk you can get this way.

- Keep expressing for as long as you are getting milk out. Switch to the second breast when the flow subsides on the first, then go back to the first one again, then the second. Better still, express from both breasts at the same time (this is possible using a pump as well as by hand—ask the hospital staff for help).

- You may want to use breast compression (see page 203) while expressing to help you get more milk.
- **Focus on putting in the order, not on what you're getting out.** Don't be disheartened if you just get small amounts to start with. It can take a little while, but the more you "ask for" the more you'll start to get. (Don't use a bigger container than you need—filling a small bowl is more encouraging than half-filling a larger one.)

tip

If you're expressing long term, you may occasionally experience a dip in how much milk you get when you express. This could be because your let-down reflex isn't working as well as it was (maybe you're worried about your baby's condition, or perhaps you've started to take the reflex for granted and have cut down on the preliminaries you use at the beginning of an expressing session), or it may simply be because you haven't been expressing very often recently. Taking your time to get ready to express and fitting in a couple of extra expressing sessions a day is probably all that's needed to boost your milk supply again. Meanwhile, you can fall back on your store of breast milk (see page 195).

After the "Wake-Up"

If you follow this approach, by the end of the two weeks you'll be producing lots of milk—possibly as much as 20 ounces per day, or even more. Of course, your baby won't need this much for a while yet, but you will have given your breasts a very clear message about what they need to do. If your baby is still not ready to have all his feedings at your breast, you'll need to keep expressing, though not quite as intensively. With a bit of experimentation, you'll find a pattern that keeps you producing milk fairly steadily. Once your baby is having most of his feedings directly from your breast, you'll be able to phase out the expressing altogether.

Hindmilk Feeding—Helping Your Baby Get More of the Fattier Milk

Premature babies can sometimes benefit from help to get more calories without having to take in more milk. If you are producing more milk than your baby needs, the NICU staff may suggest that you do something called "hindmilk feeding" so that he gets the maximum calories in the minimum of volume. At each expressing session (or feeding), your milk gets gradually creamier and more full of calories as the fat content increases. This fattier milk is sometimes known as "hindmilk." Hindmilk feeding ensures that the baby gets the calorie-rich milk first. Here's how it works:

- You express some milk from each breast (about half the amount you usually get) into one container and set it aside.
- You then express the remaining milk from both breasts into a second container. (It will probably look visibly creamier than the first batch.)
- Your baby is given the *second* container of milk first, followed by as much of the first as he needs to complete his feeding.

You may also be advised that your milk needs to be "fortified." This involves the addition of some extra minerals (e.g., calcium), usually as a powder. It doesn't mean your milk is not good quality—it's just a nutritional safety net that is thought to be important for very premature babies.

Feeding Your Baby Before He Is Ready to Breastfeed

Most babies are not mature enough to feed effectively at the breast until they reach 34 to 36 weeks' gestational age. If your baby is born earlier than 35 weeks, he is likely to need to be fed by another method for at least a short period.

WHY IS KANGAROO CARE GOOD FOR EARLY BABIES?

Kangaroo care means carrying (or "wearing") your baby next to your chest inside your clothes and is an alternative or addition to incubator care. Kangaroo care is like an advanced form of skin-to-skin contact, often with the baby secured on the mother's front with a stretchy wrap so that she can hold him and still have her hands free. Photo 11 shows a mother and baby in kangaroo care. Many NICUs encourage parents to provide kangaroo care because research shows that holding a baby this way means:

- He is less stressed.
- He has higher oxygen levels in his blood.
- He maintains his temperature better.
- He grows better.
- Bonding between the baby and his parents is better.
- His mother's breast milk production is stimulated.

Don't be afraid to ask about kangaroo care if it isn't suggested to you by the NICU staff. The more you can hold your baby like this, the better.

Feeding by Tube

Babies who are too weak to suck and swallow usually have their first milk feedings via a tube passed into their stomach through either their mouth or their nose. Neonatal unit staff are usually happy to show parents how to tube feed their babies—do ask if no one suggests it to you. If possible, let your baby have his feeding while you are holding him against your chest, so that he can smell you and feel your skin and start to associate the breast with the feeling of a full tummy.

WHY MIGHT A PACIFIER BE RECOMMENDED?

Pacifiers are often used to help stimulate digestion when a baby is being tube fed. They are also used as a way of soothing a baby who is undergoing a painful procedure, or whose parents aren't available to comfort him. Pacifier-sucking is sometimes referred to as nonnutritive sucking. Pacifiers do have a place in the care of premature babies, but they can interfere with breastfeeding if they are overused (see pages 37 and 75). Try to make sure that your baby is not given a pacifier or left sucking on one unnecessarily.

Feeding with a Dropper

Babies whose suck is weak may be able to get all the milk they need if they have small amounts put into their mouth, either expressed directly from their mother's breast or using a dropper or syringe.

Cup Feeding

Babies can lap milk from an open cup before their sucking reflex develops. Many NICUs use cup feeding for babies who don't need to be tube fed but who aren't quite ready to breastfeed. Cup feeding (see page 157) is thought to be a helpful method for premature or sick babies who are going to breastfeed later, because it happens at the baby's pace. Ask the staff caring for your premature baby whether he can be cup fed and whether staff can show you how to do it.

Bottle Feeding

Bottle feeding is the most demanding way for a premature baby to get food. Although the milk can be made to flow readily (so sucking hard isn't necessary), the baby still has to learn to stop and start the flow to enable him to coordinate breathing and swallowing. Bottle feeding is particularly unhelpful for a baby who is going to be breastfed later, because it teaches him to expect something to be poked into his mouth, which is likely to interfere with his instinct to scoop up the breast. If you *do* need to give your baby a bottle feeding, see page 156 for some tips on how to minimize the possible disruption to breastfeeding.

Helping Your Baby Move On to Breastfeeding

As your baby matures, he'll gradually move toward breastfeeding, but it's best not to rush him. As you spend time holding him skin to skin, you'll notice him start to nuzzle and lick your breast, and before long he'll begin to be able to move his head and arms, which will help him find your nipple. Expressing a few drops of milk will encourage him to search for food. It's best to avoid using perfume or scented toiletries, or even washing your breasts before offering a feeding so that he learns to recognize your natural smell.

If you focus on holding your baby skin to skin so he can breastfeed as soon as he wants to, there'll be no need for anyone to decide when he is ready for his first attempt at feeding—he'll show you by doing it.

The days and weeks before your baby begins feeding at your breast are ideal for experimenting with a few different nursing positions to help you become confident holding him in more than one way. Premature babies often have weak muscles, so they need good support for their upper back and neck. Aim to hold your baby securely, with most of his body touching you. If you're in a lying-back position with him on top of you (see page 41), all you'll need to do is steady him so he doesn't flop sideways. Upright and underarm positions can work well, but be sure not to prevent your baby from tilting his head back—just like a baby born at term, he needs to be able to tilt his head if he's to open his mouth wide and scoop up your breast at the right angle (see page 34). (See page 271 for more information on how to help babies with low muscle tone to breastfeed.)

Once your baby is showing signs of being able to feed, it's a good idea to encourage your let-down reflex before he attaches so that he won't have to make too much effort to get milk. As with a full-term baby, it's important to make sure he is effectively attached at the breast so he can breastfeed efficiently and give your breasts the right message. Stroking his face, especially downward over his nose and lips, will encourage him to open his mouth and root for your breast. Offering the breast after pumping—so it is soft and pliable—will make it easier for your baby to learn to latch. Nipple shields are sometimes advised for premature babies, but using a shield is unlikely to help your baby attach effectively—see page 39 for why.

Most women who are pumping find that one breast has a slightly faster milk flow than the other. Offering your baby this breast first each time he nurses is another good way of making sure he gets milk quickly with the minimum of effort. If your milk flows slowly, some gentle breast compression (see box, below) may help speed things up—but don't overdo it. Your baby needs time to breathe between swallows. If you have a very fast flow or are making more milk than your baby needs, expressing some milk before he starts to feed will make the flow gentler.

Premature babies aren't normally able to ask for feedings, so nursing them only on demand would be dangerous—they simply wouldn't get enough milk. In a neonatal unit, they are usually fed on a schedule that starts with hourly feeds, then moves to two-hourly, then three-hourly. (Some NICUs may still aim for four-hour gaps, which is not realistic or helpful for breastfeeding babies.)

BREAST COMPRESSION CAN HELP YOUR BABY GET MORE MILK

Breast compression is a way of increasing the flow of milk so that a baby who doesn't have much energy to feed gets plenty of milk. If, partway into a feeding, your baby is making sucking movements but has stopped swallowing, support your breast in your hand and gently close your hand around it. Apply gentle, even pressure to compress or squeeze the breast. You should notice your baby starting to swallow again. Relax your hand until he stops swallowing and then repeat the process. Be careful to use your whole hand and to avoid squeezing for longer than about a minute at a time. (If you pinch with your fingers or keep the pressure up for too long, you could stop some parts of the breast from draining properly.)

However, once your baby gets near the age when he should have been born, he may suddenly ask to nurse before his scheduled feeding is due. If you're not expecting this, it's easy to assume that breastfeeding is going wrong. In fact, he's just showing you that he's ready to regulate his own feedings in the way that full-term babies do.

Once your baby starts asking for feedings earlier than scheduled, it's time to relax the schedule and be led by him. Provided he asks for at least eight feedings in twenty-four hours (or as advised by the NICU staff), you can trust him if he chooses a longer gap occasionally. You'll know he's getting enough by his general behavior and his pees and poops (see pages 99 and 102). Before long you'll be able to relax completely, allowing him to find a pattern that ensures you carry on producing the amount of milk he needs.

Breastfeeding Twins (or More)

Being a parent of twins or triplets can be hugely demanding and time consuming, especially in the early months. Most of the practical aspects of mothering take at least twice as long when there is more than one baby. But while the practicalities of breastfeeding may take a bit of sorting out in the beginning, once you get going, it's much less effort than making up formula. It's also an ideal way to help you bond with each of your babies.

The majority of mothers can easily produce enough milk for two or even three babies, and possibly more. And despite what friends or relatives may assume, making all this milk puts no extra physical strain on the mother. Your breasts are made for the task and **if there is twice the demand, there will be twice the supply.** Breastfeeding also makes it easy to hold and nurse two babies at the same time, if that is what you want to do.

However, it's common for multiple births to have the added

complications of prematurity and/or cesarean section, both of which can make it more difficult to get breastfeeding going (see pages 62, 63, and 191), so you are likely to need extra support from your partner or family. Organizations that offer specific support with the challenges of looking after more than one baby may also be useful (see "Sources of Information and Support," page 292).

> "Most people think breastfeeding twins will be the hardest thing in the world—but honestly, once you get going, it's the easiest option. I just can't imagine making up double lots of formula and sterilizing all those bottles!"
>
> Sarah, mother of Alex, 4 years, and Holly and Jessica, 2 years

Why Bottle Feedings Won't Make Things Easier

Like all nursing mothers, those who have more than one baby need someone to help them with their other responsibilities while they come to grips with feeding (see Chapter 5). Making milk isn't tiring, but keeping up with changing diapers, washing, and dressing can be, and it's easy for those tasks to get in the way of breastfeeding.

It's common for partners or relatives to want to help mothers of multiples by offering to take over some of the feedings with a bottle. However, just as with single babies, if this happens early on, it can make things harder in the long run. While giving the occasional bottle may seem like a kindness, it's likely, in the early weeks, to interfere with the babies' learning, making effective breastfeeding harder for them. And giving them formula will reduce the amount of milk you produce.

If you want to combine formula and nursing so that feeding can be shared, it's important to allow each baby time to get the hang of breastfeeding before you introduce a bottle. This will give your babies the best chance of being able to breastfeed as well as bottle feed, and will help ensure that your breasts get a clear message from the beginning that they need to make plenty of milk. That way you'll be able to do as much or as little breastfeeding as you choose later on.

Mothers who are nursing more than one baby often find that their appetite is much larger than usual, but taking care of their own needs can sometimes be pushed down the list of priorities. Although not eating and drinking won't affect your milk supply, it may make you tired and irritable. Eating well and having a healthy snack and a drink every time you breastfeed is a good way to make sure you stay on top of things—so preparing meals and snacks for you is one of the best ways those around you can support you as a nursing mother.

How Do I Feed Two Babies?

Holding one baby for feeding takes a bit of practice; holding two is trickier again. However, there is no need to feel you have to rush to feed two babies together. Nursing them separately can give you a chance to get to know them as individuals and to find out what works best for each. All babies are unique, and it's quite common for different feeding positions to work for each baby and for them to feed at different speeds.

If you want two babies to breastfeed at the same time, lots of positions are possible. There's no need to hold both babies the same way, but you do need to make sure they are close enough to your body to tilt their head back easily to scoop up the breast, especially while you are all learning. In the early weeks, a lying-back position (see page 41) with your babies on their tummy on top of you will probably be the easiest. This way, they will have freedom to wriggle around to position themselves, and you'll have both arms free to steady them if they need it.

Whatever nursing positions you choose, you'll probably find it helpful to have someone with you to hand over the second baby once the first has started feeding. It's a good idea to start with the baby who needs the most support to latch on (if there's a noticeable difference) so you can use both arms to help him if you need to. **Once your babies have gotten the hang of feeding, managing both together will be easier.**

When you are caring for two or more babies, it can feel as though you get no time to do anything else except breastfeeding. Trying to synchronize when your babies feed can help. Breastfed babies will almost always take up an opportunity to nurse if it's offered (even if they are sleepy), so unless their feeding patterns or needs are very different, you can offer both babies a feeding whenever one asks, waking the second either at the same time or immediately afterward. (It doesn't matter if one baby feeds from both breasts and the next one feeds immediately afterward—your breasts work their hardest when they're well drained, so there's always milk available.) This strategy is definitely recommended if you are breastfeeding more than two babies.

Sometimes mothers of twins find that one baby naturally seems to prefer the right breast; and the other, the left. If they are both feeding enthusiastically and effectively, there is no reason to try to persuade them to swap sides. However, if one baby is noticeably weaker than the other, swapping sides can be a good idea. Allowing the stronger baby to put in the order for more milk on his twin's behalf—either at alternate feeds, or at every feed for a day or two—will mean that both breasts get the same message. It will also mean that the weaker baby doesn't have to work as hard to eat. It's particularly important to use both breasts equally for breastfeeding and expressing if you are nursing one baby but are having to express milk for the other, as sometimes happens when babies are born early.

"The twins were different at the breast. I had very fast flow on my right boob, so Jenny usually had that one because she was bigger. Haley couldn't handle it, so she had the left breast, which had more normal flow. And they were different to get started, too; Jenny always latched on really well, but Haley took ages."

Sam, mother of George, 4 years,
and Jenny and Haley, 2 years

KEY POINTS

- Breast milk is especially important for babies who are born prematurely—and their own mother's milk is most valuable of all.
- Expressing intensively in the first two weeks is the key to meeting your premature baby's needs long term.
- Skin contact and kangaroo care help premature babies thrive and encourage milk production. They also allow the baby to show when he is ready to move on to breastfeeding.
- Careful choices of early feeding methods can help smooth the transition to breastfeeding for premature babies.
- Most mothers can produce enough milk for two, three, and even more babies. More demand = more supply.
- If you are planning to combine nursing with bottles, wait until breastfeeding is easy for you and your babies before you introduce a bottle.
- Multiples often have a preference for one breast or feeding position and feed at different speeds.
- Encouraging your babies to nurse at roughly the same times will reduce the amount of time you spend feeding.
- Swapping sides is a good idea if one baby is weaker than the other(s). This ensures both breasts are told to produce plenty of milk.

12

Your Milk Supply

BABY-LED BREASTFEEDING MAKES managing your supply easy. Understanding what controls how much milk you make, and the part your baby can play in changing that, is the secret to avoiding or overcoming most milk supply problems. It's even possible to start breastfeeding several weeks after your baby's birth, to go back to it after a break, or to nurse an adopted baby. This chapter looks at how to manage your milk production to meet a variety of challenges, as well as ways to reduce your milk supply safely if you have to stop breastfeeding early.

How Milk Production Is Determined

The number of milk-producing cells women have varies enormously (see box), but how rapidly an individual mother makes milk at any particular time depends on how many of her cells are working and what they are being "told" to do (see Chapter 2). The number of *functioning* cells is determined in the first few weeks. The more **F**requent, **E**ffective, **E**xclusive, on **D**emand, and **S**kin to skin the breastfeeding is (see page 71), the more cells will be activated and the greater the amount of milk the mother will be able to make for her baby (the system is reset with each pregnancy). Cells that have been primed like this can step their rate of production up or down, working more or less hard according to how much they are asked for. This is what determines how much milk the mother is actually making at any one time.

Your capacity to produce milk is individual to you, but babies are individuals, too. They have different needs and feed at different speeds, so a new baby may not follow the same pattern as your last one. All this means that each mother and baby relationship is unique when it comes to making milk.

> "I think you always worry that you won't have enough milk but if they're happy and putting on weight, it must be okay."
>
> Gina, mother of Micah, 4 months

Most Mothers Can Make Plenty of Milk

Many breastfeeding mothers worry about how much milk they are producing. Often, these concerns stem from their babies' behavior, which may not be connected with feeding. **It's extremely rare for a mother not to be able to make enough milk to feed her baby— when it does happen there is almost always a medical problem that accounts for it** (see page 218). Yet many mothers stop breastfeeding unnecessarily in the early months because they believe they can't make enough milk.

SUPPLEMENTING WITH FORMULA WON'T HELP

If you think you may not be producing enough milk, don't be tempted to give your baby supplements of formula. They will fill her up so that she takes less breast milk, with the result that your milk production slows down even more.

YOUR CAPACITY FOR MILK PRODUCTION

Almost all women can produce enough breast milk for at least two babies. The number of milk-producing cells each woman has varies—and it has nothing to do with the size of her breasts. Some women naturally have only a small number of milk-producing cells, so each cell needs to work fairly hard most of the time. These mothers need to nurse their babies very frequently to keep their milk production going at an adequate level. Other women naturally have lots of milk-making cells and struggle to keep their supply *down*. They can break all the breastfeeding rules (by feeding by the clock, using pacifiers, and so on) and still maintain a good level of production. Most mothers are somewhere in the middle.

Many common concerns, such as a fussy baby, frequent feeding, wakefulness at night, slow weight gain, and only being able to express small amounts, are assumed to indicate a lack of milk, but none of these is a reliable sign that the baby isn't getting enough. For example, wanting to nurse frequently is normal for a breastfed baby, while fussiness and crying can have many different causes. Even if the baby is currently not getting all the milk she needs, this doesn't mean her mother isn't capable of producing enough.

Almost all mothers produce plenty of milk for their baby in the first week or so, but this doesn't continue if the milk isn't removed effectively and frequently. If your baby is not spending enough time at the breast, or not feeding efficiently when she is there (or both), your breasts will soon stop producing the milk she needs. This doesn't mean your milk supply is running out or drying up—just that your baby hasn't been putting in a big enough order.

Provided your milk production was kick-started with lots of

effective feeding (or expressing) in the first few days (see Chapters 5 and 11), the capacity for you to make lots of milk is always present—you just need to tell your breasts that more is wanted. However, if you didn't get the chance to nurse your baby or express your milk early on, how much you can increase production may be limited (see page 21). It's still important, though, to help your breasts start making more milk than they have been by increasing the stimulation you give them now.

NOT ENOUGH MILK—A WESTERN PROBLEM

In communities where it's usual for babies to be close to their mother's breast 24/7, a baby will help herself to a few sucks every twenty to thirty minutes. Not having enough milk is almost unknown in these societies. In the United States, most babies have to ask for feedings, so they tend to nurse much less frequently. For many women, breastfeeding their baby fewer than eight to ten times a day means they will struggle to meet her needs.

If You Think Your Baby Isn't Getting Enough Milk

If you suspect that your baby may not be getting enough milk, start by checking the signs that breastfeeding is working. As explained in Chapter 6, her pees and poops will provide the best clues (as long as she is having only breast milk—no water, formula, or other food), followed by her behavior and weight. There are four likely scenarios:

1. **If your baby is peeing and pooping normally for her age and is gaining weight,** it's likely that she *is* getting enough

breast milk. If she just seems to be nursing very frequently (and has always done so), this is probably her natural pattern. If she's unsettled and needing to nurse more frequently than usual, maybe:

- She's going through an appetite (or "growth") spurt (see page 116).
- She's teething or coming down with a cold.
- She's feeling the need for extra comfort (is anything going on in the household that could be upsetting her?).
- Her natural nursing pattern is changing as she grows older.

2. **If your baby is peeing and pooping normally but *not* gaining weight**, this suggests she *is* getting enough milk but that she has another health problem. It would be advisable to get her checked by your doctor.

3. **If your baby is producing lots of watery, green poop and is very miserable (or colicky)**, she may be feeding in a way that means she gets the wrong balance of sugar and fat. See page 104 for how to remedy this.

4. **If your baby is not producing normal amounts of pee and poop (and isn't gaining weight) but seems otherwise well**, the most likely problem is that she *isn't* getting enough milk. See below for what to do to improve her intake.

If your baby isn't getting enough milk, it's probably related to the way she's feeding. For a baby under two weeks old, adjusting the attachment may be all that's needed, but if there's still a problem, it's likely to be that she's either not nursing often enough or is coming off the breast too early. If in doubt, remember, more **FEEDS** = more milk (see page 71). If your baby is older than two weeks, it's likely that your milk production will have started to slow down, so the problem may take a bit longer to resolve. Either way, here's how to help her get more milk:

- *Check your baby's attachment at the breast* (see page 48). **This is the first thing to do, because the rest won't work if she isn't able to feed effectively.** Is her chin indenting your breast? Is her mouth open wide and are her cheeks full? Can you see or hear her swallowing frequently? If not, you may need to hold her in a slightly different way so that she can tilt her head back more or come to the breast at a different angle.

- Unless there are serious medical concerns about her wellbeing, **don't give your baby anything else to eat or drink other than your breast milk.** Your breasts need to be told what her true needs are.

- *Watch for your baby's subtle feeding cues* (see page 76)—are you missing any signals that she might want to nurse?

- *Encourage your baby to feed more often.* If she's sleepy and doesn't seem interested, try expressing a few drops of milk on to her lips to tempt her. Holding her skin to skin may help awaken her instincts.

- *Make sure your baby is close to you at night* so she can nurse as soon as she stirs.

- *Avoid using a pacifier,* which could stop your baby (and you) realizing that she needs to nurse.

- If you've previously been taking her off the breast when you think she's had enough, **let your baby feed for as long as she**

wants on each breast. If she's feeding effectively, she *will* let go when she's had what she needs.

- *Always offer your baby the second breast* (but don't worry if she doesn't want it).

In most cases, more frequent breastfeeding (with effective attachment) is all that's needed to enable a baby to get more milk. However, if nursing has not been going well for more than a week, your milk production may have slowed down significantly. In this case, the best way to turn things around is to give your breasts a boost by following a plan of intensive breastfeeding or expressing (or a combination of both). The next section explains how to do this.

Giving Your Supply an Intensive Boost

This concentrated feeding plan should quickly get your breasts working hard and producing lots more milk. You'll need to do this if you think your milk production has been low for more than a week. It's a miniature version of the babymoon described in Chapter 5. Here's how it works:

- If possible, arrange for someone else to be around to take on your usual responsibilities so you can focus on breastfeeding.
- Find somewhere safe, warm, and comfortable where you can stay in skin-to-skin contact with your baby while you are awake (your bed or the couch, for example). This is your "nest."
- Keep plenty of drinks and snacks within arm's reach, so you don't have to keep getting up.

- Stay in your "nest" as much as you can and encourage your baby to have *lots* of feedings—*at least* one every two hours, but more often if she's willing. It doesn't matter if they are very short—the more often she feeds, the more your breasts will be stimulated to make milk.
- If you can't encourage your baby to feed at least every two hours, try switch feeding whenever she *does* nurse (see box) and express your milk between feedings.
- Continue to nurse as often as you can throughout the night.

If your baby isn't interested in nursing frequently, expressing between feedings will make sure that your breasts are given a big enough order to make more milk. However, it's important not to offer the expressed milk to your baby unless she really seems to need it, because a full tummy may stop her wanting to nurse again soon. (If you have already started giving her some formula, see page 227 for how to phase this out as your milk supply improves.)

HELPING A SLEEPY BABY GET MORE MILK

"Switch feeding" is a short-term measure that can help a baby who tires quickly to get more milk. If your baby falls asleep after only a few minutes at the breast, moving her to the other side will wake her up a bit and encourage her to start feeding again. It will also trigger a new let-down reflex, which will help her get more milk without too much effort. If she falls asleep again, switch her back to the first breast. Feeding by feeding, if she is effectively attached, she'll start to nurse for longer on each side and you'll find yourself having to switch her less often. Within a few days, you'll be able to stop switching altogether.

REMEDIES THAT *MAY* HELP YOU MAKE MORE MILK

Galactogogues are medicines, herbal remedies, and teas that can help boost milk production. However, they don't replace the need to feed or express frequently, and most have only limited evidence to support their use. In the past, mothers whose babies were in a NICU were often prescribed drugs to increase their milk supply. However, recent evidence suggests that the sort of intensive boost described above is much more likely to bring about a significant and lasting increase in milk supply than taking medications. If you *do* decide to take medicines or herbs, make sure they are prescribed by a licensed practitioner.

How Can I Tell That I'm Making More Milk?

As always, your baby's pees and poops are the best guide to how much milk she's getting (see page 99)—more out means there must be more going in. As she begins to take more milk, her behavior will change, too. If she was fussy and crying, she will start to be happier and may ask to nurse less often. However, if she was a very quiet, sleepy baby, she will probably start to be more wakeful and eager to nurse.

If your baby is under two weeks old and her attachment at the breast was the main cause of the problem, you will probably find that your breasts now feel noticeably less full after nursing. If she's older, and your milk production had gone down, you may begin to feel full before feedings again.

If you don't start to see changes in your baby's behavior and an improvement in her pees and poops within forty-eight hours, seek help from someone skilled in helping with breastfeeding (see "Where Can I Get Help?," page 108).

Less Common Reasons for Low Milk Production

Although low milk production can usually be fixed with minor adjustments to the way you breastfeed, there are some other possible causes. The first two are the most likely culprits.

- The contraceptive pill (especially the combined pill), contraceptive implants, and hormone-based coils (intra-uterine system, or IUS) can interfere with your hormone balance and reduce milk production. Tell your doctor or practitioner that you are breastfeeding before you decide to use one of these methods.
- The presence of placental fragments that have been left behind in the womb can trick your body into thinking you are still pregnant. If your tummy is tender, if you are passing bright red blood more than four days after the birth, or if you have a smelly vaginal discharge, contact your midwife or doctor as soon as possible.
- Some common medicines can be a problem. Decongestants can decrease milk production and antihistamines can make a baby drowsy and cause her to ask for fewer feedings. If you need to take medication, check that it won't affect your milk production (see pages 138 and 264).
- Smoking and drinking alcohol have been shown to have a *small* effect on the amount of available milk, but this is negligible if feeding is baby led.
- Some babies who are premature or have physical problems may need help to feed effectively (see Chapters 11 and 15).
- A very few women have a condition that may reduce their ability to produce breast milk, such as polycystic ovary syndrome or an underactive thyroid gland.

Could I Be Making Too Much Milk?

Although it's a less common concern than not having enough milk, women who produce too much milk can find breastfeeding difficult. If you are producing more milk than your baby needs, your breasts will probably be uncomfortable for much of the time. They are likely to leak a lot, and if they are very heavy, they may cause backache. The flow of milk may make your baby feel as though she is drowning during feedings. She may clamp her jaws together or pull away to try to stop the flow, or come off the breast coughing and spluttering. She may also show signs of colic (see page 103). It's easy for mothers (and their families) to interpret this behavior as being due to not enough milk or milk that isn't strong enough to satisfy the baby, but this is not the case.

Am I Really Making Too Much?

If you suspect that you are producing too much milk, it's important to make sure this is true before doing anything to tackle it. Many of the signs mentioned above can have other causes. For example, during the first few weeks it's normal for mothers to make more milk than their baby needs and for babies to struggle with the rush of milk at the beginning of a feeding. And because this is when long-term milk production is being set up, it's important not to do anything to suppress milk production during this time.

Even after the first few weeks, other causes for what appears to be too much milk are possible: Breasts can feel overfull because they are not being drained effectively; some mothers have a very strong let-down reflex or readily leak milk, even though they are producing normal amounts; a baby can show colicky behavior for all sorts of reasons, including not being effectively attached at the breast; and some babies with muscular or neurological problems (see Chapter 15) have difficulty coping with even a relatively gentle flow of milk.

To be sure that the likely cause of the problems you are experiencing is that you are producing too much milk, check the following:

- Your baby was not born before 37 weeks of pregnancy.
- She is over three weeks old.
- She is healthy and developing normally.
- She is gaining weight well (or very fast).
- She is fussy most of the time and asking to feed very frequently.
- She is passing lots of urine and watery, green stools.
- She always attaches effectively at the breast (see page 48).
- Your breasts feel full most of the time.

If any of these *don't* apply, or you are unsure whether your baby is attaching effectively at the breast, speak to someone skilled in helping with breastfeeding (see "Where Can I Get Help?," page 108) before doing anything to reduce milk production. If you are in any doubt about your baby's general health and development, see your doctor first.

"I always had a lot of milk—I'd have to change my breast pads every time I changed a diaper and I was always leaking. I just thought it was normal. As soon as he latched on, Alfie used to pull away spluttering and milk would squirt all over him. At ten weeks he started getting green watery poops that 'fizzed' and every evening he'd have terrible colic. And he was hungry all the time. It settled down a bit when he was about six months, and it wasn't until after that—when I was looking through a breastfeeding book for something else—that I realized I'd had oversupply. I had no idea there was anything I could have done."

Sara, mother of Alfie, 5 years

What to Do If You're Making Too Much Milk

A mother who isn't producing enough milk can feed her baby more frequently to increase her supply, but as someone who is making too much milk you can't just cut down the number of feedings your baby has. Your milk is digested as fast as any other mother's and your baby's stomach can only hold so much at one time, so she will still need to nurse fairly frequently. But that doesn't mean there's nothing you can do to make things easier for you both.

Mothers who have a tendency to overproduce can easily get into a vicious cycle that works like this:

- The mother produces more milk than her baby can manage at a feeding.
- The baby feeds well but gets filled up before she reaches the creamiest milk.
- She is hungry again very soon because she didn't get many calories.
- Her mother's breasts get overstimulated by the frequent nursing and *increase* milk production.
- The baby gets filled up even earlier at each feeding. She is colicky—and both she and her mother are miserable.

Most babies of mothers who are making too much milk don't need both breasts every time they feed, and letting your baby nurse from just one side may be all that's needed. If the other breast feels uncomfortable, express some milk—just enough to relieve the discomfort. Leaving milk in the breasts helps slow down production (see page 23), so after a day or two you may not need to express. Using each breast only half as often may be enough to keep your milk production at a reasonable level.

If your baby is using only one breast each time she nurses and you still have a problem, the answer may be to express a small amount of milk beforehand, so that she doesn't have to wade through so much low-fat milk before she gets to the creamier stuff. That way she'll get a smaller, higher-calorie feeding, which will cure her tummy-ache and stop her needing to feed again quite so soon. Less frequent nursing will gradually encourage your breasts to slow down production. You'll need to use trial and error to find out how much to express—start with just a few teaspoonfuls and see if that's enough to make your baby happier. When your breasts start to feel less full between feedings, you can try nursing her without expressing first, to see if your strategy has worked. Many women who overproduce find that expressing a small amount of milk before each feeding for a day or two every few weeks is enough to keep the problem under control.

The "clear-out" method is a more radical solution. This involves pumping as much milk as you can from both breasts in one session. Then, at your baby's next feeding, you offer her just one breast—and keep offering that one whenever she wants to nurse during the next three to four hours. (If she comes off that side and seems to want more, you can offer her the other one, but it's unlikely this will happen if your overproduction is extreme.) Then you switch to the other breast and restrict her to that one for the next few hours.

This approach may seem strange (and it isn't exactly baby led) but it works by resting each breast in turn, which stops them from constantly refilling. And, because they start fully drained, engorgement is unlikely. Many mothers who've used the clear-out method find they can go back to a normal breastfeeding pattern after four or five days. Others find they need to stick to a one-side-for-three-hours rule indefinitely. Usually, though, the clear-out doesn't need to be repeated.

REMEDIES TO SLOW DOWN MILK PRODUCTION

There are medicines and herbal remedies that can help reduce milk production (sometimes referred to as antigalactogogues). If your overproduction isn't controllable by the methods described, you may want to consult a doctor, herbalist, or lactation consultant to see if he or she can suggest something that will help. (As with any other medications, make sure they are prescribed by a licensed practitioner and that it's safe for your baby to have your milk while you're taking them.)

Starting Breastfeeding When You Haven't Just Given Birth

Breastfeeding usually starts soon after a baby is born, but sometimes it doesn't begin until sometime later. This may be because the mother didn't want to breastfeed initially but then changed her mind, or it may be that she wants to restart after a break. Sometimes a mother wants to breastfeed an adopted baby, or one born to a surrogate mother. All of these are possible, although the level of milk production achieved varies enormously, depending on the circumstances. In each case, the individual woman's determination to make it work and the support of those around her are key factors.

If you want to start breastfeeding in one of these situations, it's a good idea to talk to a breastfeeding counselor or lactation consultant, who will be able to help you develop a personalized plan based on the following principles.

Starting Breastfeeding Late

It's never too late to decide to breastfeed your baby. However, the longer the gap between the birth and getting started, the less likely it is that you'll reach full milk production. If it's only been a week, the likelihood is that you'll be able to establish breastfeeding very quickly and you may not need to follow all the steps described below. If it's longer than that, you may have to work a little harder. In some cases, full breastfeeding won't be possible but partial breastfeeding, with some formula feedings, almost certainly will. **The information in this section will also be relevant for you if things didn't go well in the early days of breastfeeding and your baby is now having formula for some or all of her feedings.**

In the first few weeks after birth, if a mother's milk-producing cells sense that milk isn't needed, they start to shut down. Once this happens, they can't be reactivated until her next pregnancy. How quickly the shutdown happens varies from mother to mother, and unfortunately, there is no way of telling, in the days and weeks after the birth, how many milk-making cells are active. The only way to find out how much milk you can make is to give it a try.

When beginning breastfeeding some time after your baby's birth, or recovering from a difficult start, you are likely to be faced with two challenges: getting your breasts into milk-making mode and persuading your baby to feed from them. If your baby is happy to latch on to your breast, she will be able to put in most of the order for milk herself. However, if she has never breastfed effectively, she may take a while to figure out what to do. In that case, you will need to rely mainly on expressing to get your breasts working. Once they are producing more milk, persuading your baby to latch on will be easier.

There are three main ways to get your breasts to start making milk:

- *Giving your supply an intensive boost* is the quickest and most effective method. See page 215 for how to do this.
- *Waking up your breasts gradually, over a week or two* (see below) may suit you better if you want to take things more slowly.
- *Using a nursing supplementer* (see page 226) is a gradual alternative but it can be awkward, so it's not ideal for short-term use.

Here's what to do if you want to wake up your breasts gradually, so they return to milk making over a period of a week or two:

- Offer your baby the chance to nurse as often as you can (don't wait until she's hungry). Hold her so she can nuzzle against your breast when she's drifting off to sleep or just stirring awake.
- Hold your baby skin to skin as much as possible. This will help her feel safe and happy near your breast and stimulate you to release the hormones you need to make milk. If possible, carry her skin to skin in a sling so you can continue to hold her even when you need your hands free for something else.
- Massage your breasts and nipples and hand express between feeding opportunities.

The following will help persuade your baby to breastfeed:

- Hold your baby next to your breast when you're bottle feeding her. If you can, express a little breast milk and smear a few drops over the bottle nipple before you offer her the bottle to help her associate feeding with the smell of your breast milk.

- When you're offering your baby a bottle feeding, brush the bottle nipple down over the tip of her nose and her top lip to encourage her to tilt her head back, open her mouth wide, and reach forward with her tongue—as she will need to do at the breast.

Once your baby is nursing frequently, watching her behavior at the breast (and especially her swallowing; see page 94) will give you clues as to how much milk she's getting and help you figure out when to start phasing out her formula feedings.

FEEDING YOUR BABY WITH A NURSING SUPPLEMENTER

A nursing supplementer is a bottle with a fine tube that is taped to the breast so that the tip extends to the tip of the nipple. The bottle is filled with either formula or expressed breast milk. The baby takes the tube and the breast into her mouth when she feeds, stimulating the breast to make milk while she gets milk from the tube.

A supplementer allows a baby to have feedings of expressed breast milk or formula while being nursed at the breast. It can be used to help a mother relactate (see page 228) or start or boost milk production for a baby who isn't able to take much from her mother's breast directly. If long-term supplementation is needed, it can provide an alternative to bottles. A breastfeeding specialist will be able to discuss with you the pros and cons of supplementers and show you how to use one.

How to Phase Out Your Baby's Formula Feedings

As your breasts start to produce milk and you can see your baby swallowing while she's nursing, you will be able to start reducing the amount of formula she has. You can do this by giving gradually smaller amounts at each feeding over a period of several days or weeks—or you can go for a more rapid changeover, like this:

- Give your supply an intensive boost (see page 215), setting up your "nest" with drinks and snacks on hand and focusing on having plenty of skin contact with your baby—and *lots* of nursing (as often as every half hour, if your baby is willing).
- Offer your baby a bottle feeding only when she is no longer content to feed at the breast. If possible, get someone else to give that feeding so that your baby associates you solely with nursing. Don't try to persuade her to finish the bottle.
- Go back to your "nest" with your baby and continue with skin contact and lots of breastfeeding.

This approach will boost your milk production very quickly, so that breastfeeding can take over from most or all of the formula feeding within two or three days. It will also save you having to calculate how much formula to give.

Whichever method you choose, you will need to keep an eye on your baby's pees and poops, throughout and for at least a week after you stop giving formula, just to confirm that you're producing enough breast milk for her. Don't expect her feeding pattern to be the same as it was, though, especially if she was sleeping for a long period overnight; breastfeeding is meant to happen frequently, day and night.

If you don't seem to be able to get rid of the formula feedings completely, you've probably found your maximum milk production level. In that case, you can decide when is the most convenient time of day (or night) for your baby to have the formula she still needs, so that you can continue to breastfeed her frequently the rest of the time. (Tip: Don't assume that the obvious time to give formula is going to be at night; breastfeeding is usually quicker and simpler than preparing a bottle and will help both of you get back to sleep quickly—see page 116.)

Can I Produce Milk After a Break from Breastfeeding?

Sometimes mothers who have breastfed their baby in the past want to start again after a break. This is known as relactation. In some countries, it's not unusual for a grandmother to relactate so she can help feed her grandchild. In the United States, it's more usual for it to happen when a mother who has stopped breastfeeding changes her mind. If the period of breastfeeding was very brief or difficult, the situation will be more similar to starting breastfeeding late, and you can relactate using any one of the three possible approaches described on page 225.

Restarting milk production is easier the shorter the gap since breastfeeding stopped—but it's never too late. It just takes more commitment the longer you've left it.

Can I Breastfeed an Adopted Baby?

It is possible to breastfeed an adopted baby (or your own biological baby, born to a surrogate mother), but how easy you will find it, and how much milk you will be able to make, depends on your breastfeeding history, on how old the baby is when you take over her care, and on whether she has nursed before.

If you have previously fully breastfed one or more babies,

even if it was a long time ago, you will in effect be relactating, so your chances of achieving full milk production will be quite high. However, if you haven't breastfed before—and especially if you've never been pregnant—then you will be inducing lactation rather than reactivating it. In this case, full breastfeeding may not be possible.

It may be that your main aim in choosing to breastfeed is to provide your baby with your breast milk, perhaps for specific health reasons. Or it may be that what you want most is to be able to nurture her at your breast because of the emotional closeness this will bring. Your best course of action depends on which of these matters most to you.

If you want to produce as much breast milk as you can, then—ideally—you will need to start stimulating your breasts to produce milk several months in advance. Some specific methods for inducing lactation have been developed, which include a prescribed course of hormones, followed by a combination of drugs or herbal medicines and intensive breast stimulation and expression. If you want to follow this sort of protocol, we suggest you contact a lactation consultant (see "Sources of Information and Support," page 292). If you don't want to go to these lengths, you can do an extended version of the two-week "wake-up call" described on page 195 instead. Expect it to take a couple of weeks for milk to start to appear, and several more for production to build up.

If nursing your baby at your breast is more important to you than producing breast milk, then you may prefer simply to have lots of skin contact with her and give her formula feedings via a nursing supplementer (see page 226).

If you are lucky, your adopted baby will have been breastfed at some time in the past—possibly even right up until the adoption. However, it's more likely she will be used to bottle feeding, in which case see page 130 and page 225 for some suggestions that will help her be happy nursing at your breast. In the case of a surrogacy arrangement, you may be able to hold your baby skin to skin as soon as she's born (see page 53), in which case persuading her to accept your breast is unlikely to be a problem.

If You Need (or Want) to Stop Breastfeeding Early

This section is about stopping breastfeeding completely while your baby is under a year old and still reliant on breast milk. For information about ending nursing when your baby is older, see page 184. For information about stopping breastfeeding temporarily (e.g., for medical reasons), see page 150.

If you have decided you need, or want, to stop breastfeeding completely, and your baby is under a year old, you'll need to help her make the transition to formula feedings (see the following page). You will also need to consider how to manage your own comfort.

Stopping breastfeeding is best done gradually, for your sake as well as your baby's. If you do it suddenly, your breasts won't immediately recognize what has happened, so for a while they will continue producing milk at their previous rate. If you don't remove at least some of this milk you risk, at best, the discomfort of overfull breasts or, at worst, mastitis.

You can help your breasts wind down production slowly by cutting down your baby's feedings step by step, or more quickly by expressing your milk. Either way, you can expect milk production to take several weeks to stop completely.

How to Stop Breastfeeding Gradually

The gentlest way to switch from breastfeeding to formula feeding is as follows:

- Start by identifying the average pattern of your baby's main breastfeedings over each twenty-four-hour period.
- Replace one of these breastfeedings with a formula feeding.
- Allow your breasts two or three days to adjust their rate of milk production before dropping the next breastfeeding. Repeat this until all breastfeedings have been replaced.
- Try to avoid eliminating consecutive breastfeedings one after the other. Instead, alternate between feedings at opposite times of the day (or night), so that the gaps between the remaining breastfeedings stay more or less even.
- Aim to keep the times that your baby most enjoys nursing (commonly first thing in the morning and evenings or during the night) till last.
- Replace occasional, very brief feedings with a hug or a distracting activity, or, if she's over six months, with a drink or a snack.
- If you get uncomfortably full between breastfeedings, express a little milk to soften your breasts slightly. This will help keep you from becoming engorged and make it easier for your baby to attach when she next goes to the breast.

How to Stop Breastfeeding Quickly

To end breastfeeding quickly, simply replace all your baby's breastfeedings with formula and express your milk instead. There is no need to express very much milk at a time—just do it as often and for as long as you need to remain comfortable.

Using your comfort as a guide is the best way to avoid engorgement. If you save the milk you express (see "How to Store Breast Milk," page 154), you can give it to your baby occasionally in place of formula.

After a few days, you'll probably find that you need to express only two or three times a day, and this will be down to once a day after a week or so. However, although spontaneous leaking and fullness will disappear quite quickly, don't expect to get to a point where you can't express any milk at all. The breasts are meant to make milk, not to absorb it, and it's not unusual for mothers to be able to express milk many months (or even years) after they last breastfed.

Bottles don't have the same built-in comfort factor as nursing, so be sure to hold your baby close while you give her formula. You may find that she benefits from extra hugs and from some skin contact. (This may work better with another family member at first, so that she is not frustrated by the smell of your breast milk.)

Whether you choose a gradual changeover to formula or a rapid one, you may decide that you are happy, after all, to nurse once or twice a day (or more) rather than stop entirely. In that case your breasts will simply settle to producing the amount of milk those feedings require. You will find things work best (and that your breasts are most comfortable) if the remaining feedings are evenly spaced throughout the day—for example, at bedtime and first thing in the morning. And, of course, if you change your mind completely, you can boost your milk production again just by breastfeeding more often.

KEY POINTS

- Milk production is very flexible—especially when breast-feeding has gotten off to a good start. It can be increased or reduced, just by changing the "order."
- Some women naturally produce less milk than others, but almost all mothers can produce plenty of milk for their baby.
- A few women have a tendency to make too much milk, and there are ways of managing this situation.

- If you opt for formula feeding when your baby is born and then decide to breastfeed, you can switch over. The sooner you do so, the more likely you are to be able to breastfeed fully.
- If you stop breastfeeding and then change your mind, you can start again.
- You may be able to produce breast milk for an adopted baby or one born to a surrogate mother.
- Stopping breastfeeding before one year is best done gradually—for your sake and your baby's.

13

When Breastfeeding Hurts

BREASTFEEDING ISN'T MEANT to hurt; yet many mothers stop nursing before they really want to because they are in pain. The most common painful conditions are sore nipples, engorgement, blocked ducts, and mastitis. Mostly, these conditions can be avoided if breastfeeding is baby led, but they may still happen occasionally. This chapter looks at what causes breast and nipple pain and what to do to get breastfeeding back on track if it happens to you. (You may find it helpful to turn to the "Painful Breastfeeding: Quick Symptom Checker" on page 285 for an at-a-glance summary.)

Is It the Milk Let-Down?

If your baby is under a month old, the first thing to rule out if breastfeeding hurts is a painful let-down. The let-down reflex happens near the beginning of a feeding when the hormone oxytocin makes the tiny muscles in the breast contract to squeeze the milk down the ducts. For most women, if this is noticed at all, it's felt as a slight tingling sensation. However, some mothers experience it as a painful pinching or squeezing inside the breast, lasting up to about ten seconds.

A painful let-down is distinguishable from other types of breast pain because it tends to come on near the beginning of a breastfeeding (or between feedings, if something triggers it) and is accompanied by the baby swallowing more rapidly or by milk leaking. It happens in *both* breasts simultaneously and is often stronger in the breast that is not being fed from.

Most mothers who experience a painful let-down reflex find that it is only a problem in the first few weeks, while their body is adjusting to breastfeeding, and that it gradually becomes less painful. In the meantime, relaxation techniques—even those used during labor, such as slow breathing—can be useful. Humming or tapping your fingers to distract you from the pain can also help.

Sore Nipples—Why They Happen and What to Do

It's quite likely you'll experience some nipple tenderness in the early days while you and your baby are learning how to breastfeed. But it shouldn't last for more than the first ten seconds of each feeding—and it shouldn't still be happening after the first week. If your nipples are painful for longer than a brief "ouch" moment at the beginning of each feeding in the first week (page 36), or are sore at any time after this, the pain is almost certainly caused by either injury or infection. This sort of pain won't go away by itself, so it needs to be sorted out.

Sore Nipples Caused by Trauma or Injury

A mother's nipple can be injured when her baby isn't attached to the breast effectively. If he doesn't have a big mouthful of breast, the nipple will be either squashed against the roof of his mouth (the hard palate) or subjected to excessively strong suction—or both.

Nipples that are being injured during feedings usually start off just feeling sore, but if the problem isn't dealt with, the skin quickly gets damaged, leading to cracks and bleeding. Some women seem to be more prone to skin damage than others, but the cause of injured nipples—ineffective attachment—is the same in every case.

A crack across the tip of the nipple is caused by the nipple being repeatedly squashed during feeding. If your nipple looks an odd shape when your baby releases it, especially if it's wedge-shaped or has a white line across it, or is bluish or very pale, it's probably being pinched in a way that will lead to a crack developing.

A crack or tear around the base of the nipple happens when the nipple is repeatedly sucked backward and forward in the baby's mouth, stretching it so that the skin gives way. This tends to happen if the baby hasn't been able to draw the nipple far enough into his mouth. If you see your breast moving in and out of your baby's mouth while he's nursing, this sort of damage is likely to happen.

If a mother doesn't hold her baby close enough for him to be able to scoop up the breast and draw the nipple deeply into his mouth, it's easy for the nipple to be injured. A vicious cycle can develop if it has already been damaged and breastfeeding is painful, making the mother too frightened of the pain to bring her baby in close enough, and leading to further damage.

Damaged nipples are a sign that your baby isn't feeding effectively—which means he won't be getting as much milk from your breast as he should. As well as being a problem for both of you *now,* ineffective breastfeeding can soon start to affect how much milk you are producing, so it's important not to ignore it. See Chapter 3 for how to make it easier for your baby to feed effectively.

Occasionally, nipple damage is caused by a tongue tie (see page 38). This can be remedied fairly easily if it's diagnosed early and the baby is seen by a specialist.

Treating Injured Nipples

If one or both of your nipples are cracked, you urgently need to help your baby improve his attachment to the breast—with expert help if necessary. Unless they are infected (see page 239) your nipples won't require treatment—once they are no longer being damaged at every feeding, the cracks will heal within a day or two—but if you continue nursing as you have been in spite of the pain, the damage will get worse.

Although it may seem logical to rest a damaged nipple to allow it to heal, this will only work for a short time. If your baby's attachment isn't improved, your nipple will almost certainly get sore again as soon as he goes back to feeding from it. On the other hand, **once the attachment is right, you should find it's possible to breastfeed without pain, even from a nipple that is badly damaged, while allowing it to begin to heal at the same time**. If you can't get help quickly to change the way your baby is feeding, and feel it's too painful to continue, you'll need to express your milk (from one or both breasts, depending how sore they are) so that you don't become engorged. This will also allow your baby to continue having only your milk. But improving his attachment should be your priority.

To help your baby attach well, you'll probably need to experiment with different ways to hold him. There's a list of signs to watch for on page 48. Ask your partner, mother, sister, or a close friend to watch him feed—or watch him yourself, in a mirror. Bear in mind that different things work for different mothers and babies, so what works for a friend may not work for you.

While you are helping your baby attach more effectively, you may want to offer him the less painful breast first at each feeding, so that he is not as hungry when he nurses from the more painful side. If you're not sure how effective your baby's attachment is, or you are still in pain even though he appears to be feeding well, contact someone who is skilled at helping with breastfeeding (see "Where Can I Get Help?," page 108).

> "I found the first few weeks of breastfeeding very hard. We had lots of visitors over the first few days, and one day my nipple started to bleed as I was feeding. My friend said, 'Don't worry, that always happens—it won't do the baby any harm.' So I didn't ask for help. By the time I finally said something to a breastfeeding supporter, my nipple was so badly cracked I'd gotten to the point where I was scared to feed because of the pain."
>
> Gemma, mother of Jack, 8 months

"I'VE GOT BLOOD IN MY MILK!"

Sometimes a baby will bring up milk that has blood in it. There's no need to panic if this happens to you. If the blood looks fresh, it's almost certainly your blood, not your baby's. And it probably looks a lot more than it really is.

Swallowing blood is not harmful and it's unlikely that the blood made your baby spit up. However, bleeding from the breast or nipple is a sign that something is wrong, so it needs attention.

The first thing to do is check your nipples for signs of injury. If there is nothing obvious and your nipples don't feel sore, the bleeding is probably the result of increased blood flow and rapid development of the milk-producing tissue (sometimes known as "rusty pipe syndrome"—see also page 27). Alternatively, it may be coming from a skin tag (or papilloma) in one of your ducts.

Bleeding from increased blood flow or a papilloma should stop within a week or two of your baby's birth. If you have bleeding from within the breast that lasts more than a couple of weeks, it's a good idea to have it checked by your doctor.

Most products on the market (especially nipple creams) that claim to prevent or treat sore and cracked nipples don't actually do either, although they may make sore nipples feel a little more comfortable. If you have a very sore nipple, applying a little breast milk will do a similar job and will also help prevent infection. When you are at home, going topless will prevent friction from clothes.

A cracked nipple will be more painful if the skin is allowed to dry out and a scab forms. You can prevent this by smearing a tiny amount of USP-modified anhydrous (purified) lanolin over the crack after each feeding. (This will also help stop your breast pad or bra from sticking to it and causing pain when you peel it off.) As long as you keep the amount small, there's no need to wash it off before your baby feeds again.

Nipple shields are sometimes suggested for sore nipples, but they are best avoided because they tend to encourage the baby to feed in a way that isn't effective. They can also rub against the nipple, causing more damage.

Sore Nipples Caused by an Infection

The two main types of nipple infection are bacterial infection and thrush (*candida*—a fungal infection). Both cause severe pain in the nipple itself. Some women experience referred pain deeper within the breast as well, but in general, deep breast pain is more usually caused by mastitis (see page 247).

Bacterial Infection

Nipples that have been damaged can occasionally pick up a bacterial infection, although this isn't very common—mainly because they're being bathed in breast milk many times a day, which protects them. If you do see pus around your nipple or coming from it, you need to consult with your doctor who will probably prescribe a course of antibiotics. It will normally be safe for you to continue to feed your baby from that breast. To avoid further damage, you'll also need to work on making sure your baby's attachment is effective (see Chapter 3).

Thrush

Some women are more prone to thrush (a fungal infection) than others, but the risk of contracting it is slightly higher if you are taking oral contraceptives or steroids, have recently had antibiotics, or your baby is using a pacifier.

Unless you have taken (or been given) antibiotics around the time of the birth (which is common in women who are group B strep positive), thrush is unlikely in the early weeks of breastfeeding. Usually, it appears out of the blue after a period of problem-free nursing. It usually starts on one breast and is quickly spread by the baby to the other breast.

The main symptom of thrush is severe burning pain, which comes on during a feeding and continues or worsens after the feeding is over (unlike the pain of damaged nipples, which immediately lessens when the baby lets go). Some women describe this as being like "bee stings" or "feeding through broken glass." Other possible symptoms are:

- shiny or flaky skin on or around the nipples
- skin that is more pink or red than usual
- itchiness around the nipples
- cracks in the nipples that refuse to heal, despite effective attachment

If you have thrush, your baby will probably be infected, too. You may be able to see white patches inside his mouth, but these aren't always visible. Some babies with thrush pull off the breast during feedings because their mouth is sore. The infection passes through the digestive system, so babies who have oral thrush often have a sore bottom as well.

Thrush doesn't mean you have to stop breastfeeding. However, you and your baby will need specific treatment. It's a good idea to pay attention to your baby's feeding technique, too, because pain (for either of you) can interfere with attachment at the breast. A simple painkiller such as acetaminophen or ibuprofen may help.

Nipple thrush can be very persistent. Treatment usually starts with an antifungal cream, but many women find they need to take an oral medication as well. It's usual to need to continue the treatment for *at least* a week. (The single-dose remedies that are sold over the counter for vaginal thrush are not effective against nipple thrush.) Your baby will need his own medication (for his mouth, and possibly his bottom). Make sure you get individual prescriptions so that one of you doesn't continue to harbor the infection and re-infect the other.

Letting your skin breathe will help discourage thrush. Choose a cotton bra—or, better still, no bra at all. If you use breast pads, choose those without a waterproof backing and change them frequently. Avoiding yeasty and sugary foods and eating plenty of live yogurt may also help prevent an attack.

Thrush can survive on washable diapers, towels, bras, bottle nipples, pacifiers, and toys. Boil whatever you can and wash the rest in hot, soapy water, rinsing thoroughly. Ironing your bra can help kill stubborn thrush spores. And make sure everyone in the family has his or her own towel until the thrush has gone. To be on the safe side, it's best not to save any breast milk expressed while you have thrush; it could reinfect your baby if it's given to him later (even if it's been frozen).

Sometimes thrush doesn't clear up (or recurs quickly) because someone else in the family has it, without knowing. If your partner or older children are kissing your baby or your nipples, or changing your baby's diaper and not washing their hands, they may be passing the infection back to you. It's worth their being checked by a doctor—and treated, if necessary.

IS IT REALLY THRUSH?

Soreness caused by ineffective attachment can easily be mistaken for thrush. Ask a breastfeeding specialist to check whether your baby is finding it difficult to attach before you jump to the conclusion that you have thrush—it could just be that you are trying to hold him in a position that he has outgrown, or if you have been using a pillow, that it's making it harder for him to attach effectively.

Other Causes of Painful Nipples

Mothers who suffer from skin conditions such as eczema and psoriasis can find that their nipples become sore while they are breastfeeding. If this is the case for you, you will need to discuss the problem with your doctor or dermatologist so that you can find a treatment that is safe for your baby. A herpes infection of the skin on or near the nipple may mean that nursing has to be suspended on that breast until the affected area has healed (see page 150 for information on how to stop breastfeeding temporarily).

Raynaud's phenomenon (also called Raynaud's syndrome), in which blood circulation to the extremities is poor, is a rare cause of painful nipples. People with this condition often find their fingers blanching, especially in cold weather—and some mothers discover that their nipples are also affected. The nipples will often look white after nursing, and the most severe pain tends to occur when the blood rushes back into them as the baby lets go. Ineffective attachment makes the problem worse because pinching the nipples forces blood out of them. There is no cure for the phenomenon itself, but your doctor can prescribe a specific drug for the pain. Keeping the breasts and nipples warm and ensuring effective attachment will also help.

Engorgement—Why It Happens and What to Do

Engorgement is the painful swelling of the breasts that follows prolonged overfullness. The breasts feel hard, they may be inflamed (red), and the skin is often stretched and shiny. **If engorgement isn't dealt with quickly, milk production will start to slow down.**

Engorgement happens if feeding is not effective, nursing is rushed or cut short, or there is a longer gap than usual between feedings (perhaps because the baby's cues to feed haven't been noticed or he slept for an unusually long time). It is most common in the early days, when mother and baby are learning new skills and the breasts are deciding how much milk is needed, and it's especially likely to happen if overfull breasts are ignored. ("Third day engorgement" is often thought to be inevitable where mothers and babies are separated in the hospital and feedings are strictly timed, but it's now known that these practices actually *cause* the problem.)

Effective attachment, frequent feeding, and making sure your baby comes off the breast by himself are the keys to preventing engorgement (remember **FEEDS**, page 71). Being aware of how your breasts feel between feedings, and offering your baby the chance to nurse—or expressing some milk—if they begin to feel heavy, will help you avoid engorgement.

The best way to relieve engorgement is to feed your baby. However, hard swollen breasts make attachment difficult. You can help him by hand expressing some milk (see page 87) to soften your breast before he nurses. If you are still uncomfortable after he's fed (or if he isn't eager to nurse), you will need to express some more milk (either by hand or with a pump) to relieve the fullness. There's no need to try to empty your breasts (breasts are never really empty, since milk is constantly being made); just express until you feel comfortable. If you want to, you can freeze the milk in case you need it in the future (see page 155). If you have an older child who is still breastfeeding, she may be able to attach more easily than your baby, so you could ask her to feed or you could ask your partner to help.

Although engorged breasts feel as though they are bursting with milk, it doesn't always flow readily. This is partly because the swelling in the breast narrows the ducts and partly because it reduces blood flow (so the oxytocin can't get through). Soaking in a warm bath or shower or putting warm compresses on your

---

YOU DON'T NEED CABBAGE LEAVES IN YOUR BRA!

An old "cure" for engorgement was for mothers to put raw cabbage leaves over their breasts, inside their bra. It's not clear how this worked, but it did seem to help. Nowadays we know it's much more important to remove some of the milk—which relieves the discomfort quickly *and* maintains milk production—than to walk around with a bra full of wilting vegetables.

breasts before nursing or expressing can help expand the blood vessels and enable the let-down reflex to work.

> "My sister got really engorged and her baby couldn't latch on. She was holding her arms away from the sides of her body—her boobs were that sore. The breastfeeding helpline said to put warm compresses on and do hand expression. She did one side and I did the other—there was loads of milk! Then all of a sudden she grabbed a breast in each hand and said, 'Wow—they're mine again!' And half an hour earlier she'd barely been able to touch them at all."
>
> Jennifer, mother of Rebecca, 8 years,
> and Nathan, 5 years

Blocked Ducts—Why They Happen and What to Do

A blocked (or plugged) milk duct feels like a small, hard lump in the breast. It's usually an irregular knotty shape, rather than smooth and round. The plug develops when something stops the milk from moving smoothly through the duct. This can be as simple as a too-tight bra or a finger pressed into the breast during nursing. It can also happen if the baby is held in a way that prevents him from feeding effectively. Holding your baby in a different position for feeding once or twice a day can help prevent ducts from getting blocked.

At first, a blocked duct is painless, so you won't notice it unless you feel for it. Then, as milk builds up behind the blockage, it will start to feel tender. If it isn't dealt with, it can turn into mastitis (see page 247), so it's not something to ignore. **If you get into the habit of having a quick feel for lumps once a day, you'll be able to deal with problems as they arise.**

Checking after your baby has nursed will give you the best picture, because breasts sometimes feel slightly lumpy just before a feeding.

Some women are more prone to blocked ducts than others, possibly because they have one or more ducts with kinks or narrow sections in them. Kinky ducts can be a quirk of nature, or they can be the result of an injury or surgery to the breast. You can still breastfeed if you have a tendency to blocked ducts; you'll just need to check for lumps frequently.

Most blockages occur inside the breast, but ducts can also become blocked where they open at the tip of the nipple. It's not clear what causes this, but it seems that a micro-thin, transparent layer of skin forms over the opening. The milk that is dammed up shows through, appearing as a white spot or blister (sometimes known as a bleb) on the end of the nipple. This type of blockage often causes an intense, sharp pain (like a pinprick), especially when the let-down reflex operates.

Wherever the blockage is, if it has been present for a while there may be a soft plug of thickened milk in the duct, similar to thick yogurt. If your baby is nursing when the duct clears, he will simply swallow the plug, but if you are expressing you'll probably see it emerge looking like a short piece of spaghetti.

How to Clear a Blocked Duct Inside the Breast

Clearing a blocked duct within the breast is usually easy and painless. You can do it by hand, squeezing the area immediately *behind* the lump gently with your finger or thumb to express the plug, or you can help your baby clear it while he's nursing:

- Find a position in which you are leaning forward over your baby, so that your breast is hanging free, away from your body. This allows gravity to help drain the milk. If possible, position your baby so that his chin (which does most of the work) is on the same side of the breast as the lump. You may need to be inventive to find a position that works—photos 13 and 14 show two examples.

- As your baby feeds, gently massage the area over the blockage with your fingertips, using small, circular movements until you can feel that the lump has gone.

How to Clear a Blocked Duct at the End of the Nipple

A duct that is blocked at the end of the nipple requires a slightly different approach because the seal needs to be broken to let the milk out. Here's how to do it:

- Sterilize a needle by boiling or by passing it through a flame; allow it to cool.
- Make sure your nipple is soft and warm. If necessary, drape a warm, wet washcloth over it for a few minutes.
- Using the sterilized needle, gently pierce the white spot and lift the seal free. As long as you're careful, this won't hurt because there are no nerve endings in the seal.
- If the plug of thickened milk doesn't come out by itself, use your finger and thumb to squeeze behind the nipple and push it forward.
- Continue expressing for a minute or two—or feed your baby, if he's willing—to be sure the blocked area is clear.

Mastitis—Why It Happens and What to Do

Mastitis usually occurs in only one breast at a time. It's an inflammation, most commonly caused by an interruption to the normal flow of milk in one section of the breast, which then becomes hot and red—and very painful. It usually starts as a blocked duct (see page 245), but this stage can easily be missed because it doesn't hurt. If it isn't cleared, milk builds up behind the blockage and starts to seep out sideways, through the walls of the ducts—in the same way that damming a river will cause it to burst its banks. The surrounding breast tissue tries to deal with the problem by sending extra blood to the area. This is what causes the heat, redness, and pain. If the milk in the affected area of the breast isn't helped to flow again quickly, the whole of the mother's body takes up the fight and she starts to feel as though she has the flu—shaky, sweaty, and achy, with a raised temperature.

Mastitis can be accompanied by an infection, which usually needs to be treated with antibiotics. Unfortunately, the symptoms are the same whether there is an infection present or not, which means it's difficult to tell right away whether antibiotics are needed. The important thing is to follow the treatment described below; if the mastitis is the noninfective type, it will usually respond quite quickly. If it doesn't, it's likely there is an infection.

Sometimes mothers with mastitis are advised to stop breastfeeding, but this is not the answer. **It's important to continue nursing to clear the affected part of the breast—and your baby is the ideal person to help with that.** There's no risk of harming him through your milk, and provided your doctor knows you want to continue to breastfeed, any medication that is prescribed will be safe. If in doubt, he or she can check online for a suitable drug (see "Sources of Information and Support," page 291).

tip

Mastitis can make breast milk taste salty. Occasionally, the first sign of mastitis is the baby pulling off the breast and refusing to feed because the milk tastes different. If your baby suddenly seems to dislike the taste of your milk, it's worth checking your breasts for lumps and redness.

What to Do If You Have Mastitis

Unless you have had mastitis before and know what to do, it's probably a good idea to consult your midwife or doctor, or a breastfeeding specialist, for support while you treat the problem. You may also want to make an appointment to see your doctor so that you have a prescription for antibiotics on hand in case you need it (see page 250). But it's important not to waste any time before starting to deal with the problem yourself:

- Warm the sore breast with a hot shower or compress—not scalding, but about the temperature you would normally use for bathing or washing.
- Encourage your baby to feed from that breast. Hold him so that he approaches your breast with his chin at the same side as the sore area, to give him the best chance of removing milk from that part. Make sure he's attached effectively (see page 48).
- If you can bear to touch the sore area, massage it with gentle strokes down toward the nipple while your baby is feeding, or put your hand flat against your breast and press slightly against that part, to help it drain.

- Encourage your baby to feed frequently from the sore breast—at least every two hours, and preferably more often. If necessary, express the milk from your other breast to keep it comfortable so you can let him concentrate on the one with the problem.
- Try to rest and have plenty to drink (water, herb teas, juices, soup). This won't have any direct effect on your breast, but it will help keep your fever down. Taking a simple anti-inflammatory medication, as recommended by your health-care provider (such as ibuprofen—or, if you can't take anti-inflammatories, acetaminophen), will reduce the swelling and redness and help reduce your temperature, too.
- If you don't start to feel better within six to eight hours, you probably need antibiotics. If you haven't already got a prescription, see your doctor urgently. Make sure your physician knows you are breastfeeding (and want to continue), so he or she can choose the best medication for you.
- Continue with the warmth, frequent feeding, and massage for a few days (with antibiotics, if you need them), until the soreness has completely gone.

"I was exhausted when I had mastitis. It was so painful, I couldn't do anything but lie on the couch and breastfeed. Arthur would nurse for much longer than usual—it was as though he knew he had to clear it. Sometimes I'd lie down and get him to feed from over my shoulder so I could get his chin near the lump. Eventually you could see the lump going down as he nursed. After that I'd get him to feed more if I ever felt my breasts getting lumpy, just to head it off."

Jemma, mother of Arthur, 5 years, and Rose, 3 years

If your baby isn't able or willing to feed frequently, your toddler (if he is still breastfeeding) may be able to help. If not, you'll need to express milk from the sore breast, either by hand or with a pump. Hand expression (see page 87) means you can locate the sore part easily (with your thumb), but some women find using a pump (on a low setting) together with gentle stroking is equally effective and more comfortable.

As well as treating the mastitis, it's important to try to discover what caused the problem. Has your baby been feeding ineffectively? Has anything been digging into your breast or squashing it, either during or between feedings? Have there been unusually long gaps between feedings recently? Finding the cause will help speed your recovery as well as prevent a recurrence.

Once the redness and pain have disappeared and you are feeling well again, you can go back to your baby's normal nursing pattern. Just make sure that he is attaching well, and check your breasts at least once a day.

If you think you have mastitis, don't just leave it and hope it will get better on its own. By not dealing with it you risk damaging your milk production—and, if there is an infection present and it isn't treated, there is a chance it could develop into a breast abscess.

Breast Abscess—A Rare Complication

An abscess is like a large boil; it develops as the result of an infective mastitis that hasn't been fully dealt with. As with mastitis, the affected area of the breast will be hot and red, but it will also have what feels like a smooth, hard, round knob inside. This is because the pus that's produced can't drain and builds up in a sort of pocket. Breast abscesses are rare, but they are usually *extremely* painful.

What to Do If You Suspect a Breast Abscess

If you think you have an abscess, see your doctor urgently. He or she will almost certainly prescribe antibiotics and refer you to a breast surgeon to have the abscess drained (this may need to be done more than once).

If the abscess isn't too close to your nipple, and you can bear to have your baby near that breast (did we mention it's usually *very* painful?), then you may feel able to keep feeding from it while it's being treated. If so, follow the treatment for mastitis described on page 249. If you can't face it, continue nursing your baby on the other breast and express the sore one as much as possible so that you don't become engorged. (This will also help maintain milk production so that you can go back to feeding from both breasts when the abscess has cleared up.)

Once you've had a breast abscess, you are likely to have some scar tissue inside your breast. This may make you more prone to blocked ducts (and mastitis) in that breast, so you'll need to be extra vigilant about your baby's attachment and about checking for lumps, both with this baby and with any future babies.

Stopping Feeding from One Breast, If You Need To

If you are prone to problems such as mastitis but find that it occurs only (or mostly) in one breast, you can decide to stop feeding completely from that breast while continuing to feed from the other one. Most women can produce plenty of milk for their baby from just one breast, so it's unlikely you will need to introduce any formula. If possible, choose a time when you are free from your recurring problem to make the change.

You can either reduce your use of the "difficult" breast gradually or stop abruptly and express the milk instead. A gradual change will increase stimulation of the "good" breast at the same time as giving the difficult one the message to reduce production. This will keep the total amount of milk available for your baby fairly constant. If you opt for the expressing method (see "How to Stop Breastfeeding Quickly," page 231), you will need to let your baby feed very frequently from the other breast for a couple of days to increase its production. In this case, you should try to avoid giving him too much of the milk you are expressing so he still wants to nurse frequently. Unless you currently have a problem (such as mastitis) in the difficult breast, the gradual approach is probably the easiest.

The simplest way to begin a gradual changeover is to start offering the good breast first at each feeding. As milk production in this breast increases, you will be able to avoid offering the other breast at some feedings and milk production in that breast will begin to decrease. If you go a bit too fast and find the difficult breast gets uncomfortably full, just encourage your baby to feed from it once in a while, or express a little milk, until it settles down. After a couple of weeks, you'll probably find you don't need to use the difficult breast at all.

KEY POINTS

- Breastfeeding shouldn't hurt. If it's painful you need to figure out why and deal with it as soon as possible. Checking your baby's attachment is the best place to start.
- Creams and nipple shields won't prevent or cure damaged nipples—the answer is to make sure your baby is feeding effectively.
- Thrush is a fungal infection that can affect the nipples. It's easily passed between mother and baby; both need to be treated.

- Engorgement happens when breastfeeding is not effective or frequent enough—or both.
- A blocked duct is easy to detect and to treat. Checking your breasts regularly for lumpy areas (preferably after nursing) will help you avoid painful breast conditions.
- Mastitis doesn't mean you have to stop breastfeeding— and it doesn't always need to be treated with antibiotics.

14

Breastfeeding and Illness

CONTINUING TO BREASTFEED if either you or your baby is sick is important, both for health reasons and for emotional support. However, illness can make breastfeeding challenging—whether it's needing to use a different position if your baby has a cold or thinking about how to keep nursing going if one of you has to be in the hospital.

This chapter explains how to adapt breastfeeding around everyday illnesses and provides some tips for coping with more serious conditions.

Breast Milk Is the Best Food If Your Baby Is Ill

If your baby is sick, breast milk is the best food and drink for her. It contains antibodies to help her fight infection—both the germs that are making her sick and others that might make her worse. It's also packed full of easy-to-digest nutrients. Older babies and toddlers often refuse other food when they are sick and want only breast milk. (If you have stopped breastfeeding and want to start again because your baby is sick, see page 228.)

A change in your baby's feeding pattern may be the first noticeable sign that she is unwell. Typically, she will want lots of little drinks at the breast, rather than longer feedings. This may be because:

- She is thirsty.
- She has a fever.
- She is lacking energy.
- Breastfeeding is difficult or painful (e.g., if she has a blocked nose, a sore mouth, or earache).
- She finds it comforting.

Experimenting with different positions may allow your baby to feed more comfortably. For example, an upright position will help mucus drain and may make breathing easier if she has a cold and prevent pressure on her ears if she has an earache.

If you continue to follow your baby's lead with feeding, your body will adjust your milk production to meet her needs. However, if she nurses less often than usual when she is sick, you may find that your breasts get overfull. (This can also happen in the period immediately after the illness if she has fed very frequently during it.) Expressing some milk whenever you feel uncomfortable will help you avoid engorgement and keep your milk production going at its usual rate. If your baby is under two weeks old and unable to nurse frequently because of illness, you will need to express your milk as well as breastfeed her, so that the setting-up of your milk production is not interrupted.

WHY SKIN-TO-SKIN CONTACT IS GOOD FOR A SICK BABY

Skin contact can be very comforting for a sick baby. It can also help keep her temperature stable by warming her up if she's cold and cooling her down if she's too hot. Don't be surprised, though, if holding your baby skin to skin when she's sick makes *you* feel hot—that's a sign that you're taking away some of her excess heat.

tip

A moist atmosphere can make feeding easier for a baby who has a blocked nose or sinuses, or who is wheezing. Try nursing in the bathroom with the shower running hot, or in a warm bath together. A vapor rub applied to your breast near where your baby's nose rests when she's nursing (but not too close to your nipple) can also help.

"The way I produced more milk when Dayna needed it was amazing. If she was sick she'd go off her food completely and want nothing but hugs and breast milk. There always seemed to be loads for her almost as soon as she started feeding—even when she was a toddler. As long as she was sucking, my breasts would make milk, without fail."

Barbara, mother of Dayna, 5 years

Sick babies sometimes need medicine or other treatment as well as breast milk, so it's always a good idea to get your baby checked by a doctor if she is ill—and to take her back to the doctor if she seems to be getting worse. This is especially important if she is vomiting, has a raised temperature or a rash, is wheezing, or seems lethargic.

What If My Baby Is Vomiting and Has Diarrhea?

Gastroenteritis is rare in babies who are fed solely on breast milk. Breastfed babies are *meant* to produce lots of runny, yellow stools (see page 100), and while her poop may occasionally have a slightly different smell or color, as long as your baby is her usual self, this isn't a cause for concern. However, if her pooping pattern is different from usual and she is vomiting (as opposed to spitting up—see page 82), then she may have a stomach infection.

Vomiting and diarrhea can quickly lead to dehydration, so it's important to get your baby seen by a doctor. However, breast milk will probably be all she needs to allow her body to get rid of what is irritating it and replace the fluid that is being lost. Keeping an eye on how many pees she's doing will help you monitor how well hydrated she is (although this may not be easy if she is passing lots of watery poop).

Babies don't need any extra water when they have an upset tummy. Breast milk contains plenty of water, especially when feedings are short and frequent. Very short feedings are more likely to keep vomiting at bay than larger feedings, and nursing your baby in a position that makes it easier for her to control the flow of milk (see "If Your Milk Flows Too Rapidly for Your Baby," page 80) can help, too.

Animal milks (e.g., cow's, goat's, and sheep's milk) can irritate the stomach lining, so the usual advice is to avoid them—and products based on them, such as infant formula—if the stomach is already inflamed. This doesn't apply to breast milk. Human milk is gentle on the stomach, and it contains important growth factors to help the gut repair itself. In some cases, a special replacement drink (called an oral rehydration solution, or ORS) may be prescribed in addition to breast milk, but there is no need for breastfeeding to stop. Even when a baby needs intravenous fluids, she can usually continue to drink breast milk.

What If My Baby Needs an Operation?

If your baby needs surgery, her nursing will probably be disrupted—either just during the operation, or possibly for quite a bit longer.

If the surgery is planned, it's a good idea to visit the unit where your baby will be cared for so you can talk to the head nurse or your physician in advance. For example, you'll probably want to find out whether you'll be able to sleep next to your baby and whether there are facilities for you to express and store your breast milk on site. Pediatric ward staff don't always have much experience of breastfeeding, so you may need to explain what you need in some detail.

If your baby needs an anesthetic, ask the staff how late her last breastfeeding before the operation can be so that you can make sure you offer her the chance to nurse as close to it as possible. Breast milk passes through the stomach very quickly (and is a nonirritant), so it's usually allowed nearer to the operation than formula or any other food.

If the operation is a minor procedure, breastfeeding may be able to continue uninterrupted. If there has to be a slightly longer than usual gap between feedings, expressing some milk will stop you getting overfull. On the other hand, a long, complex procedure with complicated aftercare may mean that breastfeeding isn't possible for several days. In that case, expressing your milk will be very important, both to provide your baby with milk, if she needs it while she is recovering, and to maintain your milk production until she can start nursing again. See page 150 for information on expressing milk during a temporary break in breastfeeding.

Worrying about your baby won't affect how much milk you produce, but it can temporarily affect your let-down reflex, so your milk may take longer than usual to start to flow. This means that if you are expressing, you may need to help the reflex to work (see page 152). If you have been able to express some milk in the days and weeks beforehand and freeze it at home, you'll have it to fall back on if necessary. Just knowing it's there will help make the situation less stressful.

Breastfeeding is an effective pain reliever, especially where short-term painful procedures are concerned. **Research has shown that babies are soothed by being held, by skin-to-skin contact, by sweet tastes, and by sucking. Breastfeeding combines all of these.** Just one word of caution, though: If your baby needs to have repeated painful procedures (such as blood tests), it may be best to breastfeed her immediately *after* the procedure rather than during it, just in case she starts to associate breastfeeding with pain and begins to refuse the breast (see page 105).

If your baby can't be picked up or is unable to move easily— perhaps because she has an intravenous line or is in traction—you'll need to be inventive about how you feed her. As long as you can offer her your breast in a way that enables her to scoop it up effectively (see Chapter 3), it doesn't matter how you achieve this. Don't be afraid to ask for help from a staff member and to move furniture and use cushions to help you get close to her at an angle that will work.

Parents of very sick babies sometimes feel powerless to help their baby when she is in the hospital, especially if she needs specialized care. Continuing to nurse your baby in this situation means you will be helping her in a way that no one else can—giving her the best nourishment she can have, and comforting her in a unique and special way.

> "Saba needed heart surgery when she was eight months old. She wasn't able to breastfeed for a few days afterward so I had to express some milk. I'd never had a problem expressing before but I could hardly get anything. I think all the stress

affected my let-down. When she came home, I relaxed a bit and we had lots of hugs skin to skin and frequent feeds, and it was soon sorted."

Shazia, mother of Jamal, 6 years,
and Saba, 4 years

Can I Keep Breastfeeding If I'm Ill?

Breastfeeding mothers are often advised—by family and friends, and sometimes by health professionals—to stop breastfeeding if they become sick. Sometimes this is because of unfounded fears about passing on the illness through the breast milk, and sometimes it is in the mistaken belief that producing milk drains a mother's energy and will make her illness worse. However, there are very few situations in which stopping breastfeeding is either necessary or a good idea.

Breastfeeding reduces stress, boosts a mother's immunity, and stabilizes her metabolism. **Breastfeeding women sleep better and get more nourishment from their food than do women who are not breastfeeding, and they recover more quickly from common illnesses.** There are only a very few illnesses that can be passed on through nursing, and these are quite rare (HIV, for example, can sometimes be passed via breast milk). So continuing to breastfeed is normally in the interests of both the baby and her mother. If in doubt, consult your physician.

What If I Have an Infection?

Most common infections, such as colds and tummy bugs, are passed from mother to baby through touching, kissing, and breathing on each other, not through breastfeeding. And, while formula can become contaminated as it's being prepared, this can't happen with breast milk. If you have an infectious illness, your baby will already have been exposed to the germs that caused it before you know you are sick, so by continuing to breastfeed you will be protecting her from it—or helping her get better, should she catch it.

In the case of some infections—chicken pox, for example—it can be advisable for the baby to be given an immunization, but there is no reason for a mother who has chicken pox (or shingles, which is related to chicken pox) to stop breastfeeding.

Sometimes a mother who is sick simply feels too unwell to continue nursing. However, it's important to bear in mind that stopping breastfeeding suddenly can lead to engorgement or mastitis (see Chapter 13), and although expressing will help prevent this, it may prove more awkward and difficult than continuing to nurse. It may be more helpful for someone to help you breastfeed your baby than for her to be given a bottle.

Breastfeeding Can Help with Postpartum Depression

There is a widespread assumption that mothers who have postpartum depression (PPD) shouldn't breastfeed. This seems to have arisen either because some people believe that breastfeeding makes PPD worse or because they think depressed mothers need to be relieved of the "burden" of feeding their baby. Neither of these beliefs is true. In fact, breastfeeding *reduces* the chances that a mother will develop PPD—and if she does become sick, continuing to breastfeed will make some aspects of the illness easier to cope with.

Postpartum depression can make it hard to enjoy your baby or feel close to her; it can also make sleeping difficult. Breastfeeding can help with both these problems. The hormones released during breastfeeding will promote bonding and help you relax, so although you may have to feed your baby more often—during the day and at night—you are likely to feel more rested and closer to her if you keep nursing than if you switch to formula.

However, postpartum depression can make it difficult to tune in to your baby, which may mean that you don't always spot her feeding cues, especially if they are very subtle. You may also find it hard to pay attention to how effectively she is feeding when she's at the breast. If you have a supportive partner, close friend, or family member, he or she may be able to help you make sure your baby is breastfeeding effectively and frequently.

If you are finding mothering difficult, nursing may be a key way of helping you feel that you matter to your baby, because it's something that only you can do. And if you have postpartum depression, helping you continue breastfeeding is one of the most valuable things your partner, family, and friends can do—for you *and* your baby.

"I started getting postpartum depression when Jacob was about five months old. Everything was overwhelming, and I felt inadequate as a mom. But I never lost my bond with Jacob—I didn't feel distanced like some moms who have it. I think nursing was really important for that—it was comforting for me as well as him. In a world where everything was turned upside down, breastfeeding seemed to anchor us."

Ruth, mother of Jacob, 3 years

The majority of drugs for postpartum depression are safe for nursing mothers to take. However, your doctor may want to prescribe medications that he or she believes are particularly effective but that are not recommended during breastfeeding, and advise you to change to formula so that you can take them. It may help to have a supportive partner, friend, or relative with you to help you explain why it is important for you to carry on breastfeeding and to urge your doctor to choose an alternative drug.

What If I Need to Take Medication?

Most medicines are safe to take while breastfeeding (see page 138). For the few that aren't, an alternative is usually available. However, some groups of drugs are almost always unsafe for breastfeeding babies. They include drugs for the treatment of cancer (chemotherapy). Radioactive compounds, injected for use in X-rays, can also be harmful. In some cases it is not safe for the mother to feed or even hold her baby for several hours after the procedure, until the radioactivity has worn off.

If you are told you need to undergo an X-ray involving the use of a radioactive compound or take a drug that is not safe for your baby, try to find out whether it can be postponed, if only to allow you to stockpile some breast milk in advance. If you will be able to resume nursing after the procedure or course of medication, you'll need to express to keep yourself comfortable (and to keep your milk production going) while you can't breastfeed. See "What Happens If I Need to Leave My Baby for More than a Day?," page 150, for how to do this. See "Sources of Information and Support," page 291, for some useful websites on drugs in breast milk.

What Happens with Breastfeeding If I Have to Go to the Hospital?

Keeping your baby fully breastfed while you are in the hospital isn't easy but it can be done—provided none of your drugs or treatments makes your breast milk harmful for your baby. Nonemergency admissions are obviously easier to manage than emergency ones are because they allow you to express and freeze some milk and discuss your needs with the hospital staff in advance.

Try to find a hospital that will allow your baby to spend as much time with you as possible (or negotiate more time), so that she can have at least some feedings directly from your breast. For the rest, you will need to express your milk for her, either by hand or by pumping. The hospital should be able to supply you with a breast pump, if you need one. Alternatively, you can search online for your nearest pump rental station. Make sure the fact that you are breastfeeding is recorded in your hospital notes.

If you are going to have an operation, aim to feed your baby or express your milk as close as possible to the time you go to the operating room to minimize the discomfort of very full breasts afterward. Make sure that all the doctors involved in the operation (including the anesthetist) know you are breastfeeding, and ask them to ensure that any drugs they give you are safe for you to take. Unless they tell you otherwise, it will be okay for you to nurse your baby as soon as you are awake, provided someone is there to help you hold her.

KEY POINTS

- Breast milk is the perfect food for your baby if she is sick. It contains antibodies to fight infection, it's easily digested, and it won't irritate her tummy.
- A change in your baby's normal nursing pattern can be an early sign that she is sick. Sick babies often want to have lots and lots of short feedings.
- Skin-to-skin contact can be helpful in regulating your baby's temperature.
- If your baby has an ear or chest infection or a cold, you may have to change your usual feeding position to make it easier for her to nurse.
- Frequent, small feedings will help prevent dehydration if your baby is vomiting or has diarrhea.

- If your baby needs an operation, try to plan ahead so that you can express and breastfeed while she is in the hospital.
- If you are sick, continuing to breastfeed will benefit both you and your baby.
- If you have postpartum depression, nursing can help you sleep better and enjoy your baby.
- Some situations and drug therapies mean breastfeeding has to be interrupted, but they rarely mean it has to end.
- If you need to be in the hospital, talk to the staff about having your baby with you. If possible, express some milk in advance so that you have it in reserve.

15

Conditions That Make Breastfeeding Difficult

SOMETIMES PHYSICAL OR medical conditions can make breast-feeding extra challenging, but it's very rare that it can't happen at all. Whatever the circumstances, you and your baby still have most, if not all, of the basic abilities and instincts for breastfeeding to be baby led, even if you can't use all of them in quite the same way. While it's important for you both to have help with the things you can't do, it's just as important that neither of you is prevented from doing the things you can.

This chapter looks at how conditions such as cleft lip/palate, low muscle tone, cardiac (heart), and breathing problems can affect a baby's ability to breastfeed and suggests ways to help you and your baby work around the difficulties. (For more on the effects of illness, drugs, and surgery on breastfeeding, see Chapter 14.)

Helping Your Baby Get Milk Easily

For many babies with a physical or medical problem, breastfeeding is ineffective. This means it's tiring for the baby and may not provide enough stimulation for his mother's breasts. If your baby has a weak suck, as well as helping him breastfeed as effectively as he can (see page 34), you may need to express after and/or between feedings to ensure that your breasts make plenty of milk. This will help him get milk with the minimum of effort while ensuring long-term production. "How to Give Your Breasts a Two-Week 'Wake-up Call'" on page 195 will help you maximize the stimulation you give your breasts when expressing.

Breastfeeding If Your Baby Has a Cleft Lip/Palate

A cleft lip and cleft palate can occur singly or together. Sometimes there is a cleft in the gum as well. Either condition can present a real challenge because it interferes with the way the baby attaches to the breast and how efficiently he can suck. However, even if full breastfeeding is not possible, there are several reasons why babies with a cleft benefit from some breastfeeding and from being given breast milk.

Babies with a cleft palate have an opening in the roof of their mouth, so that the mouth and the nasal cavity are connected. This means they often get milk leaking into their nose while they feed; breast milk is much less irritating to the lining of the nose than formula. They are also prone to ear infections, which breast milk can protect against. Breastfeeding helps strengthen the muscles of the upper lip and palate, which will promote healing after surgery and aid eating and speech development later.

Surgery to repair a cleft lip is usually carried out while the baby is quite young. Breastfeeding is normally possible as soon as the effects of the anesthetic have worn off. There is no risk to the stitches from nursing, although the area will probably feel tender at first. Surgery to repair a cleft palate is not usually carried out until the baby is a few months old. A palatal obturator is sometimes fitted before this, to help prevent the cleft from closing unevenly, but these are of only minimal help with feeding. It can be challenging to keep breastfeeding going until surgery is possible, so it's a good idea to ask for all the support you can from friends and family.

If Your Baby Has a Cleft Lip

Having a cleft lip interferes with the baby's ability to form a seal around the breast. If there is no seal there will be only limited suction, so breastfeeding will be inefficient and tiring. A small cleft may be able to be filled by the breast, provided it's not too full and can mold itself to the shape of the baby's lip. Breastfeeding your baby frequently and expressing some milk before nursing, if necessary, will help keep your breasts soft and pliable. If the cleft is too big to be filled by the breast itself, you may be able to use your finger or thumb to seal the gap while he feeds. Experimenting with different feeding positions will help you find what works best for you both.

If Your Baby Has a Cleft Palate

The cleft may be in the soft palate, the hard palate, or both. A cleft palate causes problems for breastfeeding in three ways:

- The cleft prevents a seal from being formed around the breast within the mouth, so suction is limited.
- Milk can leak into the baby's nose during feeding.
- If the cleft involves the hard palate, there may not be a firm surface for the baby's tongue to press the breast against.

In addition, babies with a cleft palate are inclined to hold their tongue in the cleft and to be reluctant to stretch it forward to scoop up the breast. A palatal obturator may help, but in general, full breastfeeding for a baby with anything other than a very small cleft is not likely to be possible. In that case, you will be shown how to use a specially designed bottle and nipple to give your baby supplementary feeds.

The following tips will help you maximize your baby's effectiveness when feeding at the breast:

- Experiment with your breasts being either firm or soft during feeding to find out which suits your baby best. Expressing some milk will soften your breast; using breast compression (see page 203) will make it firmer.
- Experiment with nursing positions. Holding your baby so that his head is higher than his chest will help prevent milk from leaking into his nose—for example, lying back with him on your tummy, or sitting upright with his legs straddling your thigh. (If you have a long back, you may need to use pillows to raise him to the right level.)
- If your oral surgeon suggests fitting a palatal obturator, ask for one with a smooth surface to help avoid trauma to your nipples.
- Experiment with support for your breast and/or your baby's jaw to help him keep the breast deeply in his mouth. The "Dancer" hand position (shown below) may help.

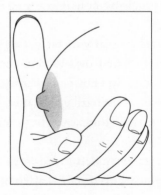

To support your baby using the "Dancer" hand position:

- Cup your hand under your breast, so that your last three fingers and part of your palm are supporting your breast and your thumb and forefinger are free.

- Open your thumb and forefinger to make a U shape. Bring your baby to your breast so that his chin rests in the center of the U. Touch the pad of your forefinger to one of his cheeks and the pad of your thumb to the other.
- Continue to support his jaw with gentle pressure on his cheeks throughout the feeding. Take care not to prevent his jaw from moving up and down.

Breastfeeding If Your Baby Has Low Muscle Tone or Heart or Breathing Problems

Babies with weak muscles, a cardiac (heart) condition, and/or breathing problems tend to have difficulty nursing, either because their jaw and tongue movements aren't effective or because they tire quickly. Yet breastfeeding is particularly valuable for these babies because of the protection it gives against chest infections and because it is less disruptive to their breathing and heart rhythms than bottle feeding.

Breastfeeding is particularly valuable (but often dismissed as too difficult) for babies with Down syndrome, because it protects against immune system and bowel problems, to which they are prone, and strengthens the facial muscles and tongue, providing long-term benefits for eating and speech.

Babies whose muscles are weak or who lack energy need to be able to feed without too much effort. Nursing in an upright or semi-upright position will help your baby coordinate swallowing and breathing. It's important to provide gentle support for his head while still allowing him to tilt it backward. It helps some babies maintain their attachment at the breast and suckle more effectively if gentle pressure is applied with a fingertip just under and behind their chin in a rhythmic, scooping movement, or if their lower jaw is supported using the "Dancer" hand position (see page 270).

Breastfeeding can't be entirely led by a baby who tires easily, since he's likely to need encouragement to feed. Stimulating his rooting reflex by stroking his face, especially his nose and lips, will encourage him to open his mouth. Patting his lips gently with your finger before putting him to the breast may also help. Holding him in skin contact while he is asleep will mean you can move him toward your breast as soon as he begins to stir, helping conserve his energy for feeding.

A nursing supplementer (see page 226) may help your baby get more milk for the same amount of effort. Alternatively, if he is not able to feed effectively at the breast, you will need to express after nursing and give him the milk using a dropper or small feeding cup. Babies with breathing or heart problems may also benefit from "hindmilk feeding" (see page 198) to help them gain weight.

> "Breastfeeding is like everything else with Down syndrome babies—it takes longer for them to learn and you need to be extra patient and put in more effort. It was challenging in the beginning because Rana was so sleepy, but it got better. It's worth it. She breastfed until she was two and she was always really healthy when she was little. I'm sure that was due to nursing."
>
> Fahima, mother of Rafee, 10 years,
> and Rana, 8 years

KEY POINTS

- 🔑 Many health problems can affect breastfeeding, but they rarely make it impossible.
- 🔑 It's worth seeking skilled, expert help from a breastfeeding specialist if you are facing a situation that will make breastfeeding unusually challenging.

Conclusion

OUR AIM IN writing this book has been to provide you with practical information that will enable you and your baby to establish a happy and harmonious breastfeeding relationship and avoid the all-too-common problems that spoil the experience for so many families. We hope it has given you the knowledge and confidence to take a baby-led approach to breastfeeding, helping you and your baby develop a strong and lasting bond.

The quick reference section that follows summarizes some of the key information from the book. It includes the essentials of baby-led breastfeeding, what to expect as breastfeeding progresses, and a quick symptom checker to help you track down the reason if you are finding breastfeeding painful.

We hope you have enjoyed this book, and we wish you and your baby a rewarding and relaxed breastfeeding experience.

Quick
Reference

Baby-Led Breastfeeding— In a Nutshell

BABY-LED BREASTFEEDING RELIES on you and your baby being in tune so you can respond to her needs and she can help your breasts make plenty of milk. If she's allowed to nurse whenever she asks, you will be able to keep pace with her need for milk as she grows. However, it's important that she's able to attach effectively each time so that she can get milk easily and give your breasts the right messages. This will also ensure nursing is pain free for you.

In a nutshell, aim for breastfeeding to be:

- **Frequent**—day and night
- **Effective**—with your baby attached so that she can get milk easily
- **Exclusive**—your baby has only breast milk—no other drinks or food (for the first six months)
- On **Demand**—whenever your baby asks, and for as long as she wants each time
- **Skin to skin** as much as possible in the early weeks

Here's how to do it:

1. **Get to know your baby's feeding cues so you can feed her before she gets upset.** Offer her a feeding *before* she asks, if your breasts are uncomfortably full.

2. **Get reasonably comfortable before nursing, but don't make your position too fixed.** Have a small cushion or a rolled-up sweater ready in case you need it. A snack and a drink is a good idea, too.

3. **Hold your baby in a way that will make nursing easy for her,** with:
   - as much of her body in contact with yours as possible
   - her whole body in line (with her knees and nose facing the same way)
   - her body weight supported (neck, shoulders, and hips)
   - her head and arms free
   - her nose lined up with your nipple ("nose to nipple"). Support your breast, if you need to.

4. **Give your baby time to attach and start feeding.** Help her by bringing her in *really* close, very quickly, when her mouth is at its widest (unless she's lying on top of you, in which case she'll do it herself). Make sure you don't have your hand on her head as you do this.

5. **When she starts to feed, check that:**
   - Her chin is pressed into your breast.
   - She has a wide-open mouth.
   - Her cheeks are full and rounded.
   - More of your areola is showing above her top lip than below her bottom lip (if you can see any of it).
   - She is starting to suck in a rhythmic way, with a big yawning movement followed by a swallow.

6. **Decide what you need to do to be comfortable.** For example, use a cushion or rolled-up sweater to support your elbow or back. Relax and enjoy nursing your baby.

7. **Let your baby feed for as long as she wants.** When she lets go of the first breast, offer her the second. Be ready to offer her the first again afterward if she seems to want it.

When she turns down the chance to reattach, that's when she's had enough.

Breastfeeding this way will help you make as much milk as your baby needs and ensure nursing is comfortable and relaxed.

Baby-Led Breastfeeding: What to Expect When

IT'S A GOOD idea to know what to expect as breastfeeding progresses, so you can either be reassured your baby is behaving normally or quickly spot any potential problems. If you think your baby is unwell, or you are struggling to care for him, contact your midwife or doctor. If you want specific help with breastfeeding, you may prefer to contact a breastfeeding specialist (see "Where Can I Get Help?," page 108) or support organization (see "Sources of Information and Support," page 290). The following table outlines what you can expect, provided you and your baby are well.

WHEN	WHAT TO EXPECT— YOUR BABY	WHAT TO EXPECT—YOU	WHAT TO DO	SEEK HELP IF...
First few hours	1 to 2 hours awake and alert, then a long sleep. Will find the breast on his own and have his first feeding. Note: Wakefulness may be delayed if drugs are used in labor.	Exhausted but not sleepy (at first). Ready to get to know your baby.	Have uninterrupted skin-to-skin contact, at least until your baby has nursed for the first time.	—
First 5 days	Number of feedings per day increasing, peaking on day 5. Gradually more pees. Poop changing from dark green/black meconium to runny yellow mustard (see page 99). Small weight loss—no more than 10%. Mild jaundice may develop from day 2.	Breasts gradually feel heavier as milk production gets going. May feel let-down reflex as tingling; possibly some leakage. Milk changing from thick yellowish colostrum to whiter, less concentrated milk. Some nipple tenderness possible at the beginning of feedings. After-pains while nursing. You may be emotional and weepy ("baby blues") from day 3.	Keep your baby near you, day and night. Encourage your baby to nurse frequently, especially if you feel full. A lying-back position can help you both learn. Watch and listen to him feeding; notice his sucking and swallowing pattern. Learn to express your milk by hand.	... breastfeeding hurts beyond the first few seconds of a feeding. ... your baby doesn't swallow after every 1 or 2 sucks. ... your breasts are engorged. ... your baby isn't peeing more each day. ... your baby's poop isn't changing color.

WHEN	WHAT TO EXPECT— YOUR BABY	WHAT TO EXPECT—YOU	WHAT TO DO	SEEK HELP IF . . .
5-14 days	Jaundice gradually fades (usually by day 7 or 8). Nursing frequently—probably 12 times or more in 24 hours; may be erratic. Birth weight regained. Frequent yellow poops.	Breastfeeding is pain free. Breasts feel full before feedings and softer afterward. "Baby blues" lessen.	Keep your baby near you day and night. Encourage your baby to nurse frequently. Give only breast milk. Avoid bottles and pacifiers. Experiment with different nursing positions. Learn to breastfeed lying on your side. Get into the habit of checking your breasts for lumpy areas once a day.	. . . breastfeeding hurts. . . . your breasts are hard or lumpy. . . . your baby isn't feeding at least 6 times a day. . . . your baby isn't doing at least 6 pees and 2 poops each day.
2-6 weeks	Baby's own nursing pattern emerging. Nursing 6-12 times a day (or more)—cluster feeding likely. Gradually becoming more adept at breastfeeding. Poops may be less frequent from 4 weeks.	Breasts feel full before feedings and softer afterward. Need to concentrate less when nursing.	Keep your baby near you day and night. Offer your breast whenever your baby asks (or earlier). Give only breast milk. Avoid using a bottle until confident your baby is breastfeeding effectively. If you want to use a pacifier, keep use to a minimum.	. . . breastfeeding hurts. . . . your breasts have a hard, red, or lumpy area. . . . your baby isn't feeding at least 6 times a day. . . . your baby isn't doing at least 6 pees and 2 poops each day. . . . your baby is still jaundiced.

WHEN	WHAT TO EXPECT— YOUR BABY	WHAT TO EXPECT—YOU	WHAT TO DO	SEEK HELP IF...
6 weeks– 3 months	Feedings may become shorter (as breastfeeding gets more effective). Occasional "appetite spurts" likely. Beginning to smile and communicate in new ways. May be long gaps between poops.	Breasts start to feel soft most of the time (unless there is an unusually long gap between feedings). Breastfeeding starting to be something you can do without concentrating.	Keep your baby near you day and night. Offer your breast whenever your baby asks (or earlier). Give only breast milk. If you want to use a pacifier, keep use to a minimum.	...breastfeeding hurts. ...your breasts have a hard, red, or lumpy area.
3–6 months	Gradually more interested in surroundings. May not want to focus on nursing. Occasional "appetite spurts" likely. Possibility of teething.	Breastfeeding is second nature.	Keep your baby near you day and night. Offer your breast whenever your baby asks (or earlier). Give only breast milk. If you want to use a pacifier, keep use to a minimum.	...breastfeeding hurts. ...your breasts have a hard, red, or lumpy area.
6–9 months	Interested in handling and tasting solid foods and trying new ones; may eat small quantities. Poop may contain small pieces of solid food. Teething likely.	The occasional bite while nursing is a possibility.	Offer your breast whenever your baby asks (or earlier). Let your baby know that you don't want to be bitten (learn to intercept when it's about to happen). Invite your baby to join in your mealtimes and begin to explore solid foods.	...breastfeeding hurts. ...your breasts have a hard, red, or lumpy area.

WHEN	WHAT TO EXPECT— YOUR BABY	WHAT TO EXPECT—YOU	WHAT TO DO	SEEK HELP IF...
9–12 months	May start to nurse less frequently or for less time. Enjoying a range of foods, eating something at most mealtimes. Feeding himself efficiently with his hands. May want to try using silverware.	Milk production may begin to lessen, especially if baby has drinks of water.	Offer your breast whenever your baby asks (or earlier). Include your baby in as many family mealtimes as possible.	... breastfeeding hurts. ... your breasts have a hard, red, or lumpy area.
12–36 months and beyond	Nursing becoming less frequent—but just as enjoyable and special. Using spoon and fork with food more efficiently.	Milk production gradually declining as child feeds less often.	Offer your breast whenever your baby asks—or negotiate timings with your toddler. Continue nursing for as long as both you and your child are enjoying it.	... breastfeeding hurts. ... your breasts have a hard, red, or lumpy area.

Painful Breastfeeding:
Quick Symptom Checker

BREASTFEEDING SHOULDN'T HURT. If it *is* painful, the following chart will help you identify what's wrong and point you to where you can find more information in this book. **If you can't resolve the problem yourself, seek help** (see "Where Can I Get Help?," page 108). Bear in mind it's quite common for more than one problem to occur at the same time, especially when the root cause is the same.

WHERE THE PROBLEM IS	APPEARANCE	FEELING	LIKELY DIAGNOSIS	CAUSE	REMEDY
One or both nipples	Nipples may be slightly pink or red.	Pain at the beginning of a feeding in the breast being used	**Initial attachment not ideal, but baby quickly adjusts.**	Baby not held close enough and/or encouraged to attach before mouth is open really wide.	Pull baby's bottom in closer. Wait for wide open mouth before encouraging attachment (see page 97).

WHERE THE PROBLEM IS	APPEARANCE	FEELING	LIKELY DIAGNOSIS	CAUSE	REMEDY
One or both nipples	Nipples misshapen when baby lets go and may appear white or bluish. Otherwise, nipples red, may be cracked and bleeding.	Pain throughout a feeding, which stops when baby lets go. Nipples may be painful to touch.	**Ineffective attachment lasting throughout a feeding**	Baby being brought to breast at wrong angle, with neck or body twisted—not held close enough—encouraged to attach before mouth is open really wide, or a combination of these.	Ensure baby held close, head and body in line, nose to nipple. Wait for wide open mouth before encouraging attachment (see page 48). A lying-back feeding position may help (see page 44). Ask a breastfeeding specialist to check attachment.
One or both nipples and areolas. May be deep breast pain.	Nipples and areolas may appear pink and/or shiny.	Sharp or burning pain throughout a feeding, which continues (or worsens) when baby lets go.	**Thrush infection**	Infection with *candida*. May follow a course of antibiotics. May have been passed on by another family member.	Confirm diagnosis with breastfeeding specialist. Seek treatment for mother and baby (and possibly other family members). See page 241 for further remedies.
Both breasts (often behind the nipple)	Nipples and breasts not inflamed, damaged, or sore	Short-lived pain soon after the beginning of a feeding, accompanied by leakage of milk or sudden increase in baby's swallowing.	**Painful let-down reflex**	Rush of oxytocin causing squeezing of milk ducts. This is a normal part of breastfeeding (although not always painful).	Breathe slowly as pain peaks and subsides. Will become less noticeable after the first weeks (see page 234).

WHERE THE PROBLEM IS	APPEARANCE	FEELING	LIKELY DIAGNOSIS	CAUSE	REMEDY
One or (usually) both breasts	Breast(s) shiny and swollen. May be red. Swelling may extend into armpit(s).	Breast(s) feels hard to the touch. May have fever.	**Engorgement**	In early days: ineffective attachment and/or infrequent feeding or shortened feedings. Later: unusually long gap between feedings or stopping breastfeeding abruptly.	Feed when baby wants for as long as baby wants. Ensure effective attachment at all feedings (see page 30).
Usually one breast	White spot (bleb) visible at tip of nipple	Pain, especially while nursing. May be tender to touch.	**Blocked duct near nipple opening**	Unknown—may be ineffective attachment	Express milk plug from duct (see page 246). Ensure effective attachment at all feedings (see page 30).
Usually one breast	Small, hard lump in breast	May be pain, especially while nursing. May be tender to touch, but may be pain free.	**Blocked duct within breast**	Ineffective attachment. Pressure on the breast from tight bra, bikini top, or other clothing, or from fingers while nursing.	Ensure effective attachment at all feedings (see page 30). Try a change of position. Leaning over position may help (see page 246).

WHERE THE PROBLEM IS	APPEARANCE	FEELING	LIKELY DIAGNOSIS	CAUSE	REMEDY
Usually one breast	Hard, red area in breast, often wedge-shaped. May extend into armpit.	Severe pain, especially while nursing. May have fever. May feel shivery and achy (flulike).	**Mastitis. If problem has existed a long time, may be an abscess.**	Ineffective attachment and/or long gap or shortened feeding and/or pressure on breast from clothing or sleeping position. May involve infection, especially if nipple cracked or any pus visible.	Ensure effective attachment at all feedings (see page 30). Try a change of position. Nurse baby more on sore breast. See page 249 for more remedies. May need antibiotics; abscess will need to be drained.

Sources of Information and Support

These pages contain just a few of the many websites and online forums that will provide you with breastfeeding information and help you access support with nursing.

General Breastfeeding Information

The Academy of Breastfeeding Medicine (ABM) is a worldwide organization of physicians dedicated to the promotion, protection, and support of breastfeeding.

www.bfmed.org

The United States Breastfeeding Committee (USBC) is a nonprofit coalition of influential professional, educational, and governmental organizations with a common mission to protect, promote, and support breastfeeding.

www.usbreastfeeding.org

Baby-Friendly USA is the accrediting body for the Baby-Friendly Hospital Initiative (BFHI) in the United States. The BFHI is a global program sponsored by the World Health Organization (WHO) and the United Nations Children's Fund (UNICEF) to encourage and recognize hospitals and birthing centers that offer an optimal level of care for infant feeding. Currently, fewer than 5 percent of US births take place in a Baby-Friendly facility.

www.babyfriendlyusa.org

The Centers for Disease Control and Prevention (CDC)'s Division of Nutrition, Physical Activity, and Obesity (DNPAO) is committed to increasing breastfeeding rates throughout the United States and to promoting and supporting optimal breastfeeding practices. The CDC compiles an annual Breastfeeding Report Card and offers a Guide to Breastfeeding Interventions.

www.cdc.gov/breastfeeding

The Coalition for Improving Maternity Services (CIMS) is a group of individuals and national organizations with concern for the care and well-being of mothers, babies, and families.

motherfriendly.org

The US Department of Health and Human Services has illustrated its support for breastfeeding through the Surgeon General's Call to Action to Support Breastfeeding.

www.surgeongeneral.gov/topics/breastfeeding/index.html

The American Academy of Pediatrics (AAP) has a Breastfeeding Initiatives website:

www2.aap.org/breastfeeding

Its sister site, **Healthy Children**, also has information on breastfeeding:

www.healthychildren.org/english/ages-stages/baby/breastfeeding

Breastfeeding Law provides information on US laws about breastfeeding in public and pumping at work.

breastfeedinglaw.com

The National Conference of State Legislatures (NCSL) provides a fifty-state summary of breastfeeding laws and an overview of policy topics.

www.ncsl.org/issues-research/health/breastfeeding-state-laws.aspx

The Office on Women's Health (OWH)'s mission is to provide leadership to promote health equity for women and girls. The website has a useful section on breastfeeding, including breastfeeding in public and going back to work.

www.womenshealth.gov/breastfeeding

Work And Pump.com provides information helpful for combining breastfeeding and work.

www.workandpump.com

Practical Information and Mother-to-Mother Support

La Leche League International is a volunteer breastfeeding support network with members and groups across the US and worldwide.

www.llli.org
www.lalecheleague.org

Kelly Mom is a popular website that provides support and evidence-based information on breastfeeding, sleep, and parenting.

kellymom.com

Breastfeeding Inc. aims to empower parents by ensuring they receive the most up-to-date information to assist them with their breastfeeding baby. The site contains lots of helpful videos, many from Dr. Jack Newman's breastfeeding clinic in Toronto.

www.breastfeedinginc.ca

Breastfeeding.com has lots of information on breastfeeding, provided by a panel of experts.

www.breastfeeding.com

The Massachusetts Breastfeeding Coalition is just one of the many state-based coalitions of volunteers and experts that lead advocacy efforts and provide information and resources.

massbfc.org

Medications and Breast Milk

Infant Risk Center is Texas Tech University Health Sciences Center's information forum and telephone helpline on drugs in pregnancy and while breastfeeding. It is managed by Dr. Thomas Hale, who is considered the leading expert in this field.

www.infantrisk.com

LACTMED is part of the Toxicology Data Network provided by the United States National Library of Medicine.

toxnet.nlm.nih.gov/cgi-bin/sis/htmlgen?LACT

Collecting and Saving Breast Milk

The Human Milk Banking Association of North America (HMBANA) is a non-profit association of donor human milk banks that aims to facilitate establishment and operation of milk banks in North America. The website provides information on how to contact a milk bank to donate milk or to order donor human milk.

www.hmbana.org

Milkies sells a useful device for collecting milk while breastfeeding.

www.mymilkies.com

Special Topics and Circumstances

The Mother-Baby Behavioral Sleep Laboratory is Dr. James McKenna's website at the University of Notre Dame. It provides evidence and guidance on co-sleeping, with an emphasis on the value of breastfeeding.

cosleeping.nd.edu

Kangaroo Mother Care has information about the value of skin contact and breastfeeding for premature babies.

www.kangaroomothercare.com

Preemie Parenting shares information on the care of premature babies.

www.preemieparenting.com

The **Yahoo group APMultiples** is a useful resource for parents of twins and more.

groups.yahoo.com/group/apmultiples

The American Pregnancy Association has information on breastfeeding a baby with cleft lip/palate.

www.americanpregnancy.org/birthdefects/cleftlip.htm

BFAR has information on breastfeeding after breast and nipple surgeries.

www.bfar.org

Help with Finding a Practitioner

To find a lactation consultant:

United States Lactation Consultant Association

www.uslca.org

International Lactation Consultant Association

www.ilca.org

To find a craniosacral therapist, chiropractor, or cranial osteopath:

The Upledger Institute

www.upledger.com

The International Association of Healthcare Practitioners

www.iahp.com

Medfinds

www.medfinds.com

The International Chiropractors Association

www.chiropractic.org

You can also find supportive and skilled practitioners through word of mouth from other parents.

Further Information on Baby-Led Weaning

Our previous books on baby-led weaning (*Baby-Led Weaning* and *The Baby-Led Weaning Cookbook*), as well as the following websites may be useful, along with the growing number of parenting forums and blogs that discuss this approach to introducing solid foods:

www.baby-led.com
www.rapleyweaning.com

Acknowledgments

WE WOULD LIKE to thank everyone whose ideas, experiences, comments, and wisdom have helped create this book. They include colleagues, clients, acquaintances, and friends past and present—including those whose insights we didn't recognize for what they were at the time.

We are particularly grateful to Sue Ashmore, Claire Davis, Jessica Figueras, Emily Hussain, Hazel Jones, Wendy Jones, Derrick Murkett, Jules Robertson, Jacqui Stronach, Anne Strong, and Anne Woods for valuable feedback on the manuscript and for insight, support, and inspiration, and to Jess Fedenia and Nikki Lee for their help with adapting the text for the USA.

Thanks to Gaby Jeffs of Magneto Films for supplying some wonderful photographs, and to all the families pictured. We are grateful to them for allowing us to share their special moments.

Thanks, also, to our long-suffering editors, Louise Francis and Gill Paul, for their patience and tolerance; to Cara Bedick for her support with the US edition; and to our agent, Clare Hulton, who has believed in us from the beginning.

Finally, we would like to thank our families for their constant support while we were writing—for keeping us fed and watered, and putting up with our tantrums when things went wrong.

Photo Credits

THANKS TO THE families for permission to use the following photos (© Gaby Jeffs of Magneto Films):

Photos 3, 4, and 30: Billie, Mike, and twins Ottilie and Anna, newborn and at 8 weeks

Photos 5, 6, 14, 20–24, and 34: Roma and Artemis, 8 weeks

Photo 7: Munira, 6 weeks

Photo 11: Michaela and Jacob, 5 weeks

Photos 13, 26–28, and 31: Bronwen and Layla, 12 weeks

Photos 15–19, 25, and 32: Nadine and Beatrice, 6 weeks

Photos 33 and 36: Rachael, Valentine, and Aaron, at 2 and 4 weeks

Photo 36: Kamila and Natasha, 10 weeks

Photo 38: Tracey and Nathan, 8 weeks

And thanks to the families who provided us with these photos:

Photos 1 and 2: Clare and Scarlett, newborn (© Nick Caro)

Photo 12: Trudy, Derek, and Noah, newborn

Photo 29: Julia, Cassia, 3 years, and Fabian, 1 year (© M. Tomkins)

Photo 35: Maja and Bella, 20 months (© Cliff Castle)

Photo 37: Callista and Ivy, 6 months

Photo 39: Natalie and Jonah, 13 months (© Adam Inglis)

Photos 8–10 reprinted with kind permission from NCT's "What's in a Nappy?" leaflet, 2012 (www.nct.org.uk).

Index

About the Authors

Gill Rapley has worked as a midwife and a public health nurse. She has also been a voluntary breastfeeding counselor and lactation consultant. More recently, she spent fourteen years working for the UNICEF UK Baby Friendly Initiative, helping maternity and community health workers to implement good standards of care for mothers and babies. She and her husband have three grown-up children and live in Kent, England.

Tracey Murkett is a writer and journalist, and she is also a voluntary mother-to-mother breastfeeding helper. She lives in London, England, with her partner and their daughter, now age seven.

Gill and Tracey are the authors of *Baby-Led Weaning: The Essential Guide to Introducing Solid Foods and Helping Your Baby to Grow Up a Happy and Confident Eater* and *The Baby-Led Weaning Cookbook: 130 Recipes That Will Help Your Baby Learn to Eat Solid Foods—and That the Whole Family Will Enjoy.*

Other Baby-Led titles by Gill Rapley and Tracey Murkett
available from The Experiment

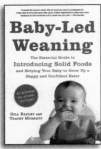

264 pages
8-page four-color photo
   insert
$14.95
Trade paperback: 978-1-
   61519-021-8
Ebook: 978-1-161519-124-6

Baby-Led Weaning
The Essential Guide to Introducing Solid Foods—and
Helping Your Baby to Grow Up a Happy and Confident Eater

The definitive text on baby-led weaning, *Baby-Led Weaning* explodes the myth that babies need to be spoon-fed, showing why self-feeding from the start of the weaning process is the healthiest way for your child to develop. With baby-led weaning, you can skip purées and make the transition to solid food by following your baby's cues.

"I recommend this groundbreaking book to every new mother I know."

—Kathleen Kendall-Tackett, PhD, IBCLC, clinical associate professor of pediatrics, Texas Tech School of Medicine

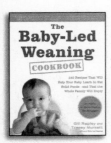

192 pages
Color illustrations throughout
$15.95
Trade paperback: 978-1-
   61519-049-2
Ebook: 978-1-61519-168-0

The Baby-Led Weaning Cookbook
130 Recipes That Will Help Your Baby Learn to Eat Solid
Foods—and That the Whole Family Will Enjoy

This companion cookbook is filled with simple advice on which foods to start with, 130 healthy and delicious recipes, at-a-glance information on nutrition, ideas for quick snacks and meals, and anecdotes from real parents. *The Baby-Led Weaning Cookbook* will give parents the confidence to create exciting and enjoyable mealtimes that will encourage little ones to develop food skills at their own pace.

"This engaging resource should match the popularity of the previous guide." —*Library Journal*